ENDERMOLOGIE®

The Missing Link Your Damaged Body
Needs for Optimal Health

THE SUPER MACHINE

FIONA SELBY

First published by Ultimate World Publishing 2021
Copyright © 2021 Fiona Selby

ISBN

Paperback: 978-1-922497-76-5
Ebook: 978-1-922497-77-2

Fiona Selby has asserted her rights under the Copyright, Designs and Patents Act 1988 to be identified as the author of this work. The information in this book is based on the author's experiences and opinions. The publisher specifically disclaims responsibility for any adverse consequences which may result from use of the information contained herein. Permission to use information has been sought by the author. Any breaches will be rectified in further editions of the book.

All rights reserved. No part of this publication may be reproduced, stored in or introduced into a retrieval system, or transmitted in any form, or by any means (electronic, mechanical, photocopying, recording or otherwise) without the prior written permission of the author. Any person who does any unauthorised act in relation to this publication may be liable to criminal prosecution and civil claims for damages. Enquiries should be made through the publisher.

Cover design: Ultimate World Publishing
Layout and typesetting: Ultimate World Publishing
Editor: Maria Joshy
Cover Image Copyright: ©LPG systems 2020

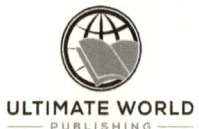

Ultimate World Publishing
Diamond Creek,
Victoria Australia 3089
www.writeabook.com.au

Testimonials

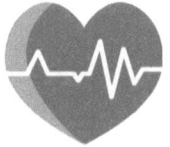

I am very grateful for all your care, expertise, information and support. I have been a client for 5 years now and I still can't rave enough about you. I trust you completely not just with myself but also all my family. I often would rather contact you before I would see my local doctor – I know I get better results. This is because you don't just treat what you see but you look for why it is there in the first place!

I constantly recommend you to all my friends and family. You are so amazing! I look forward to all my treatments and consultations.

Congratulations on all that you do and I thank you for looking after me and my family!

Thank you so much for going out of your way to accommodate me in, your very busy practice.

I really want to thank you especially for your caring and professional ways. Nothing is too big a challenge for your expertise!

Thank you for being an exceptional Naturopath.

Elisha Azzopardi

I must say to have 'Charlie' in my life is truly a game changer. endemologie® is something that not only makes you look good, it makes you feel an inner health which many don't understand. Your skin texture is firstly the biggest noticeable change, it becomes very smooth and clears away lumps and bumps along with shaping and lifting in areas we all strive for usually through exercise. Then there is the inner health of your organs, he unblocks intestines and lymph nodes, ensuring your body is operating at an optimal level no tablets or drug can provide. If teamed with the infra-red wrap, this aids Charlie's hard work in not only circulating your blood flow, but releases toxins in your body resulting in that healthy feeling and glow.

This wrap is equivalent to a 10 km run so you're sweating away fat and toxins imitating a fat loss you normally would gain from exercise while you're just lying down relaxing. I find Charlie very therapeutic, however I don't have acid build up in my muscles or huge amounts of toxins anymore, and love the feeling of release and relaxation. But wait there's more! yes, Charlie offers soooo much he also does my face and can I tell you it too has awesome results. He plumps your skin out and gives you a youthful look... let alone your lips!!! I don't know how many times I have been asked, have I done something to my lips. Yes, I have been smooching with Charlie as well, haha.

I find the expense of endermologie® far outweighs the other modern-day approaches to health issues. I am lucky I don't have any problems and at the age of 50 I feel a lot is attributed to Charlie...with menopause looking at my door I certainly don't have the issues many do at this age. Maybe it's good genes but I feel having Charlie in my life is a huge part in my success with my health, body and soul... Truly in love and addicted to Charlie (oh and the beautiful Fee as well) and she truly is the driving force behind Charlie and is an unbelievable wealth of knowledge and support in any health concerns... whether you follow her guidelines or not, with Charlie on her side, trust me you want them on your side...it is not an overnight treatment and requires a few goes but being committed to a decent block of treatments you will see results definitely. But I must warn you, it is addictive and once you get levelled up you can drop back to a maintenance of monthly treatments.

I have been committed for many years now so for me the results speak for themselves, you mean so very much to me and honestly as you can read above, I wouldn't be the person I am today without you in it...so much love for you and Charlie oh and Brandy too xxxxx so glad you have decided to live in Moranbah as you truly are loved by so many here and provide us with a service that is on another level to our wellness in living in a mining town.

Janine Madden

I was gifted with a session with Fee. Ladies big shout out if you are tired of the dreaded night sweats, struggling with the dreaded hot flushes?

Seriously Fee has the answer!

After a session with Fee I kid you not! I have had 3 hot episodes with ½ the usual heat in the last 24 hours!

Even my HRT patches weren't working!

I normally have up to 50 a day & can't cope!

Thank you Fee can't wait to see you when I get back.

Huge Thanxs!!

Cindy Taylah Barics

I cannot recommend Fee more highly. She is extremely knowledgeable, knows what works and most importantly is caring and kind to all her clients. Her treatments have made a massive difference to mine and my family's health and well-being. Thank you!!

Dee Dent

I've been visiting Fee in Moranbah on and off for six years.

Whenever I've needed a system reboot or generally to feel healthier, Fee is my go-to.

Endermologie® and happy wraps are my treatment of choice. After the first session, you can feel the difference.

Would recommend Fee and her clinic to anyone.

Miranda Taylor

Fee is amazing. My results both physically & emotionally are incredible.

I can't thank you enough for the encouragement to get me the results I wanted. Still a little way to go but soo much closer...

Netty Mouat

Feel like I was meant to meet Fee! She helped me in so many ways, and exploring my DNA was amazing!!

Sammy Walsh

I've been having treatments with Fee for several years & can highly recommend them for weight-loss, toning, cellulite reduction, fluid retention, reducing cold & flu symptoms etc.

I found the wraps amazing when I was suffering with back issues as they would ease the pain & improve my flexibility & ease of movement. Fee is a professional operator who has a great rapport with her clients and makes everyone feel at ease.

Lindy Fraser

Thanks so much for my endermologie® treatment and wrap yesterday! I had the deepest and most restful sleep I've had in years and woke up feeling so refreshed and energetic! As soon as my head hit the pillow I was out, and woke up in the same position, normally I'm tossing and turning trying to stay asleep. It was like magic. I can't wait to have more now! Also losing 1.5 kilos in one day is a bonus haha thank you soooo much!!!

Kate Paraskevos

I found Fee to be a very caring person; professional, extremely knowledgeable and accurate with her diagnosis. She is able to determine and treat the underlying cause of your problems instead of simply treating your symptoms. I highly recommended Fee to anyone.

Vanessa Cochrane

I have been a client of Fee for a number of years now. Her whole holistic and intuitive way of healing is like none other I have experienced. Her wealth of knowledge and expertise in areas of beauty, healing and naturopathy is a credit to her ongoing commitment to her clients' health and well-being. I can't recommend Fee's practise highly enough. I can guarantee one treatment, and you will be hooked on how amazing you feel and look.

Diana Donaldson

Dedication

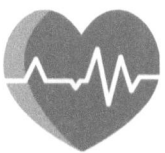

To my amazingly supportive family Manuel and Kate, Anastasia and Chris and most of all my little people, my grandbabies that light my life up with lots of cuddles, Sid, Georgie and London. Your understanding of me having to go out remote for long periods and sometimes miss out on our family times is precious. You all are my driving force and motivation to keep going and achieve my dreams.

To the people of Moranbah and the beautiful relationships, I have formed with so many people out there. Your support has been my rock in growing my successful business and making an impact on people's health. Being able to buy my clinic in Moranbah has all been to your tremendous support.

Finally, to my dear friends; Terena Blanton-Downs, we met at University and have never looked back. Thank you for pushing me through those difficult times. And to Diana Donaldson, if it weren't for you and your family, I would never have made it back out to Moranbah again to start this fantastic journey you have such a kind heart and are always there for me God bless.

Disclaimer

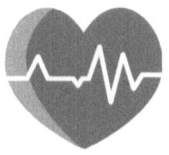

This book is written on personal experiences whilst treating clients and their results. None of the treatments can cure and do not replace medical advice. If you are unsure please seek advice from your GP immediately.

Contents

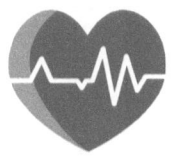

Introduction	xv
Part One: The Client	**1**
Chapter 1: Weight-Loss and Cellulite	3
Chapter 2: Anxiety and Depression	13
Chapter 3: Menopause	21
Chapter 4: Children	31
Chapter 5: Men's Health	41
Chapter 6: Thyroid	51
Chapter 7: Fertility	57
Summary: Part One	63
Part Two: The Therapist	**67**
Chapter 8: Endermologie® Machines	69
Chapter 9: Psychology in Business	79
Chapter 10: New Face Detox	87
Chapter 11: Machine Combinations	97
Summary: Part Two	109
About the Author	113
References	117
Offers	119
Speaker Bio	123

Introduction

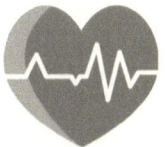

Losing weight is a mind gamer. Change your mind, change your body.
                              Myweightlossdream.co.uk

Endermologie® is the missing link, the proven treatment to look good and feel good. With this machine, it kick-starts your health physically, mentally and emotionally; and to finally find happiness in your life with the energy to achieve your goals. As I sit here on my veranda, with my beautiful dog and dedicated receptionist Brandy, in Moranbah out West of Australia, I look back on my four university degrees that I have done and realise I love all the science on health I have learnt but the real richness I have gained is from experience in treating my clients. I have now reached a stage whereas the client is walking in, by the time they get to the treatment room, I have their health all worked out and a plan in place. As a Herbalist, Naturopath and Nutritionist, my biggest challenge is getting them to make the changes in their lifestyle.

I stumbled across endermologie® when I had my first session in Sanctuary Cove in 1997 when endermologie® was new to Australia, and this was the start of my amazing journey. I had a history of obesity within my family. I realised very quickly that this was my missing link to my health, to not follow down the obesity path and for my clients in helping heal their health and to start on a fantastic journey of helping so many people throughout Australia.

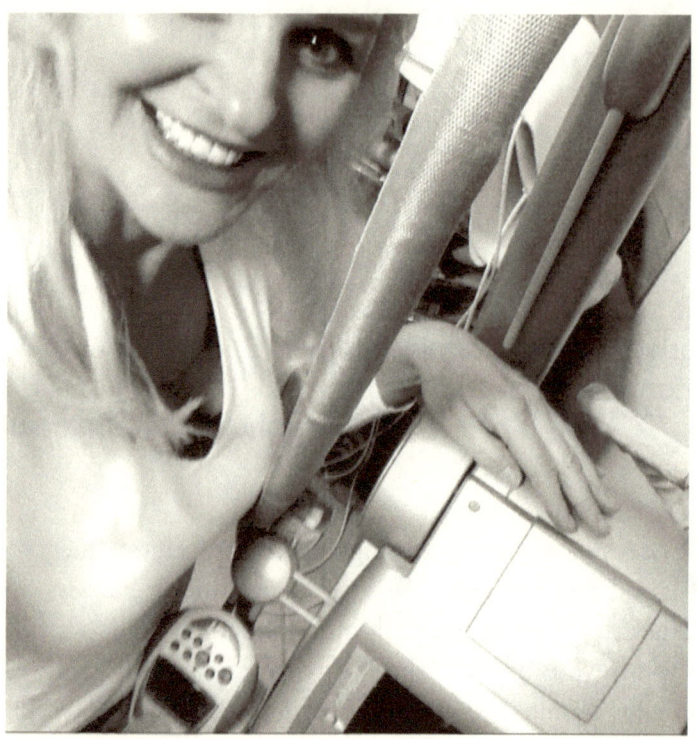

Me back in 1997 with my first machine

Endermologie® is the name of the treatment, but the machine is called Cellu M6® Alliance or 'Charlie' to all my clients. It originates from France, and the company is LPG®. I trained many years ago and have continued designing my treatments through studies and research on all my clients.

My passion for healing people came after I was driving on a country road on my way to work at Cobb n Co in New Zealand at my

Introduction

waitressing job, when I was 18 years old. Suddenly my car lost control, I still don't know why to this day. Due to 10-15 rolls, my car roof was flattened, but somehow my head had been thrown out the side window as I landed in a ditch.

I remember being sucked through a tunnel and seeing an amazing white light, the experience I had was unbelievable. It was like a flash, but it was also like in slow motion. I saw everything and understood everyone for why we are here and I was here to help heal as many people as possible and basically to stop my current life and get on with it. Suddenly I woke up to a doctor that was on his way to the hospital, pulling me out of the car. God obviously had another plan for me and sent me back.

My learning from this experience was the incredible white light and how beautiful and calming it was. From this experience, I came back with excess electricity and over the next ten years, I was a pain in the butt to live with, as anything electrical I burnt out or broke. It was an unusual experience and time in my life, but one that has stayed with me and helped mould me into who I am today. I love working with electricity and machines. Through this, I devoted myself to healing and being of service to people to help them achieve a full, happy, healthy mind, body and spirit.

I achieve my goals living in a small beautiful coal mine town called Moranbah, two hours inland from Mackay within Australia. It's a very strong community with strong family values; in other words, we have each other's backs in times of need. I have seen a house get burnt down out here and within a week that family had a home, clothes, toys and furniture provided for them. We have an amazing strong network of people that support each other out here. The land is harsh and hot with the most amazing sunsets that give me goosebumps some days. I have just bought a house here, an old miner's cottage that I am slowly renovating for my clinic. I can achieve my dreams out here of helping others to live a healthy life with endermologie® and to help keep the coal dust out of their lungs and systems. Most importantly, as I am away from my family, I can still feel part of a community… the Moranbah family.

In this book, I will be going on a deep dive into endermologie® and everything it does to help me achieve my dreams of healing others. I will be sharing in this book my experiences I learnt along my journey and how you will see a maximum outcome with minimum effort with client's health changed enormously.

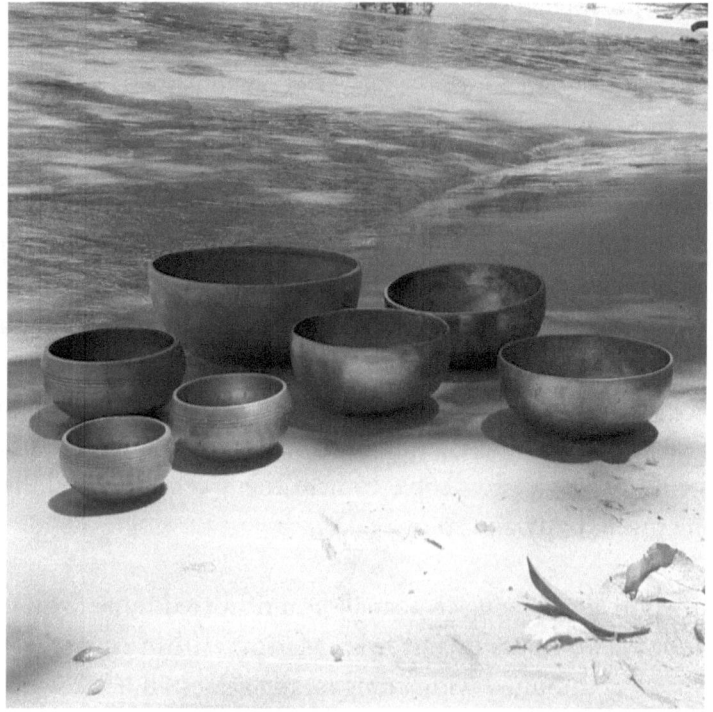

Tibetan Sound Bowls

I am also a Sound Therapist using Tibetan bowls to heal and relax the nervous system and help improve anxiety, depression or any other disease in the body that is often affected by stress, lifestyle or DNA. I was honoured to have been trained by sound masters, and from this, I have designed my unique technique to shift stuck emotion that may

Introduction

have been there for years, stuck in the body's tissues or memory brain cells, eventually affecting your health. These bowls have been used for centuries by the Monks and are very powerful. I am so excited about how powerful and relaxing these bowls are that I want to share them with you.

Please go to the back of the book to get your ***free recording*** to listen to, just before bed or when you are feeling stressed, to help relax and rejuvenate the mind. These bowls are also excellent for your child in helping them relax and sleep soundly. This ***free Sound Therapy*** recording is setting up the foundational groundwork to relax, rejuvenate and release stuck emotional junk in your nervous system and your cells.

If you find them as healing as I do, go to the free recording link in the back of the book to become a ***certified Sound Therapist*** and start your own business.

This book is broken up into two parts, the first part of the book is for you, the client …someone that has been struggling with their weight issues, thyroid, anxiety, depression, menopause, infertility or children and men's health issues.

Do you want to stop starving yourself or going on those erratic diets that you just put the weight back on anyway? Or even worse, have you got to the stage of having to have your stomach cut out where your B12 needs to be absorbed, feeling down because your life can't be enjoyed eating normal amounts of food anymore. The endermologie®, food swaps, supplements, herbal tonics and teas with the weight-loss programme does 1kg off a week, followed by the happy dance and high five, as I teach the client how to take control of their weight finally. It is an easy process and no dieting.

Are you that person that is in a stressful job, that is carrying a load of anxiety and weighing the world heavily on your shoulders with depression? Not able to socialise, difficulty walking into our Coles

Endermologie®

in Moranbah or your shopping centre without feeling the impact of social anxiety? Imagine being able to finally let go of those repetitive negative thoughts or monkey brain with the endermologie® process, designed for anxiety and depression.

Living in a coal mine town, we do get more toxicity from the coal dust. Still, it is happening everywhere; our foods aren't the same as we used to pull out of our clean soil twenty years ago, our pesticides have increased, household and personal products are full of hidden toxins. It doesn't matter where you live now; we have to include in our lives a detox regimen to relieve our bodies of toxic build-up that can cause these health issues.

These toxins affect our children, preventing our kids from reaching their full potential. They are agitated, unable to concentrate at school, angry or continually getting sick. Endermologie® is fantastic for the kids, and I will go further into our process in my chapter for children and how we can get all those hidden toxins out of their little bodies and change their behaviours.

Another popular endermologie® programme is women going through menopause. It is awful to go through, with some clients on the edge of giving up; they are so fed up with life, their jobs, their family, their partners. They are struggling with symptoms that are just crippling their lifestyles from being that happy, vibrant woman they know they can be. The constant hot flushes, mood swings and extra weight that suddenly comes from nowhere, no matter how hard they diet. This can ebb away each week as endermologie®, herbs, herbal tonics and teas bring back your womanly essence of true happiness.

Let's not forget our men that have a large gut and are always tired, in pain, exhausted, angry or even losing their testosterone. They need the endermologie® to release, unwind and let go of the build-up of toxins in their body, especially their lungs flushed due to the coal dust. Being able to promote excess blood flow for flushing the lungs,

Introduction

liver, kidneys, and lymphatic system is essential in boosting energy, improving sleep and moods.

Another area I am swamped with treating, is fertility and the toxic environmental factors and foods that are affecting our DNA, making us infertile. My years of studying DNA and needing to become an analyst in it drove me batty but now it is like my second language. Sometimes I drive my clients batty, if I start talking my DNA language, I see a haze come over their faces but the results are so worth it. My endermologie® has generations of children coming through over the years with parents and their children using endermologie®, keeping their DNA healthy and not allowing their genes to change and cause disease. I love this area the most when I have the honour to treat the whole family.

Part two of the book is focusing on the practitioner and the mechanics of the machine. But my most exciting chapter for the therapist is a newly designed Face Detox protocol that is having incredible results. It can unblock nasal, ear, throat toxins and help release clenched jaws. I have had clients that have never been able to breathe through a nostril, finally can. One client even blew their nose at the end of the treatment, and a polyp came out. There is a step-by-step guide included on how to do the new process in second half of the book.

As a practitioner and business owner, we all go through challenges and learn to adapt to new environments as we move our business around to suit our changing lives. My move out here has been so excellent. The support I have received from the community has been so encouraging, and they are always there ready to help you. If you are a practitioner, I advise that you read through all of the two parts that will help you to understand protocols I use on different health issues and the tips on how to incorporate a machine into your business. I can help you avoid the mistakes I learnt along the way and skip straight to what works best, for the most successful business where you will have a waiting list of clients wanting to see you.

Endermologie®

If you are someone that wants to know how this will help benefit you and your health, you are more than welcome to stop at the first part of the book. However, if you're like some of my test readers they couldn't put it down and went onto the second section because they wanted to know every aspect of endermologie® and the challenges faced in a remote community.

PART ONE

The Client

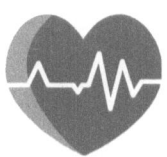

CHAPTER 1
Weight-Loss and Cellulite

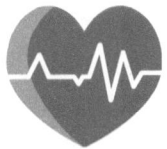

When you feel like quitting, think about why you started.
Fitspirationforlife.tumblr.com

Are you someone that has been struggling with their weight issues? Do you want to stop starving yourself or having those erratic diets that you just put weight back on anyway? Or worse having your stomach cut out; where your B12 used to be absorbed, feeling down because your life can't be enjoyed eating normal amounts of food, drinking enough water to hydrate, or finding out the emotional blockage that caused you to put all the weight on in the first place. The endermologie® weight-loss programme is incorporating components that can easily achieve 1kg off a week, followed by our happy dance when we weigh in. It is also excellent for clients in tightening the folds of skin that are left over from the weight-loss.

Endermologie®

The endermologie® weight-loss programme teaches the body to increase blood flow and circulation, preventing the fat cells from sticking together. By increasing blood flow to all your major organs in the body, oxygen is increased within the blood, causing 400% extra blood flow. This increased oxygen-rich blood can heal damage to nerves and organs, including your kidneys, liver, spleen and also improve weight-loss.

Our body can slow down from being blocked; there is such a simple solution. Endermologie® unblocks your cells from toxins that slows you down, such as coal dust clogging our systems. Having treatments motivates you to exercise and eat healthier. Don't get stuck in your funk. Break free and feel amazing.

Living in a coal mine town, lack of energy is a big issue due to long shifts and coal dust blocking our systems. Then it's hard to exercise, and with fatigue, we eat takeaway, sugar and trans-fat foods to self-medicate, to feel better but self-sabotaging our body and therefore it is common to put excess weight on.

Minerals are an essential part of our body, especially our Iron, that gives oxygen and energy to our bodies. Coal is an organic sedimentary rock that is mined by machines and breaks up into tiny particles along with crystalline silica dust particles. The coal and silica dust not only affects our lungs but also the balance of our minerals in the body.

Exposure to coal mine dust can cause various pulmonary diseases such as pneumoconiosis and chronic obstructive pulmonary disease COPD. It affects the minerals in our body causing an unbalance with crystalline silica dust particles that can get into the lungs, causing silicosis and other diseases. This is not just for the miners, but also the town people as the dust particles can travel for many miles. This causes a lack of oxygen in the blood and the lungs getting clogged.

Years ago, I was on the Fox Glacier in New Zealand hiking and was curious as to what the brown substance was on the Glazier. My guide informed me it was from the dust storms from Western Australia. I always remember this as to how far dust particles can travel.

Environmental toxins are not limited to the coal mines; it can be found on farms that are frequently around pesticides, roads with cars and the highly toxic fumes to the lungs. We are now all fighting the environmental toxins that we need to live in, and endermologie® helps you to achieve this fight. I always follow up after endermologie® treatments to check the balance of minerals and toxicity in the body through a hair mineral sample. The balance of minerals in the body is one of my favourite. After years of testing out here in the mines, the statistics I have collected show the most common heavy toxins are high Arsenic with levels that I can't even get a reading, as they are off the chart. Another common one is high Copper that causes a decline in Zinc for our immunity, causing depression, joint pain and other health issues.

I just love bringing the fundamental component of the client's health together.

As an example, too much of Copper, Sodium, Selenium, Manganese, Chromium, Nickel, Potassium and Phosphorus can lower iron levels. Or a common one is, Vitamin D when taking supplements, it helps absorb Calcium that can stop Iron absorption. There are so many more components to each mineral that can only be balanced by a trained professional. Personal supplementation can be dangerous if you are not qualified.

The endermologie® process will flush out toxins that clog our bodies up and cause weight issues from environmental pollution, leaving you feeling lighter and more energised. I use a method with the rollers that run over the lungs, just gently tapping and knocking off built-up mucus. It also helps to break down lumpy blockages in the gut to help promote healthy bowels.

I had a lady come to see me that had weight issues. I found out her bowels were releasing only once every three weeks due to her toxicity that had built up in her system over the years and she was depressed. Endermologie® was able to get her system working together to release her bowels daily. Her whole life changed; she was happier and dropped weight so quickly after that. It also helped relieve her depression and taught her body to poop again. Sometimes our body will just stop working and get lazy, and endermologie® will come in and kick it into gear.

I often have clients come to see me with excess mucus in the lungs from bronchitis, pleurisy and pneumonia. The antibiotics are just not working and they are finding it hard to breathe. One treatment instantly opens up the lungs, gently tapping the mucus and breaking it up, followed by the infra-red straps to get straight into the lungs

To do the treatment, you will wear a grey/white body stocking called endermowear™ to help prevent pulling on hair or skin being pinched and also for the client's modesty. I avoid the white body stockings as some clients have coal dust embedded in their skin. As soon as I start the treatment, the client relaxes with the action of using the rollers that roll in and roll out. The roll-in action picks the fat up and cracks it while the roll-out action drains it away and tones and tightens the skin. This process of drawing and toning the skin is important, as we sculpt the body and get into the areas that the gym or exercising can't move and we need to firm the skin after, as the fat drops away.

Cellulite

Popular areas to do are the fatty areas on the legs. I have clients that train every day but still have thickened portions. As I run the rollers down the legs, we can feel the lumps and blockages breaking up and popping like rice bubbles and draining away, to get the gap between the legs to make the legs slimmer and smoother. It's so important to break these lumps and blockages up; they stop your blood circulating freely throughout the body, slows the lymphatic system, causes blocked arteries and less blood flow to the heart. They also can cause that orange peel look, called cellulite that is stubborn to move even with exercise.

Cellulite can be hideous, its lumpy dimpled flesh that is in women and men and I'm sad to say children as well. Cellulite can be because of your genes, body fat percentage, age and the actual thickness of your skin. It can get into the thighs, hips, buttocks and stomach area. It's a fatty deposit just beneath the skin. The connective tissue has fibrous connective cords that attach the skin to the underlying muscle, with the fat lying between. What happens is, as the fat cells increase, they push up against the skin, while the long fibrous cords pull down. This creates an uneven surface and gives the dimpling effect.

What the endermologie® machine does is rolls fat cells up into the rollers, cracks them and stretches the connective cords at the same time to make them firmer and tighter causing the skin to tighten, tone and smooth out, getting rid of that dimpling effect. The result is your skin feels silky smooth; it's like having a face-lift on your body, getting rid of dimples and that crepey, ageing skin.

The Gut

Another popular area to break up is the gut. The main area is the shelf I often get from women having babies where fatty tissue forms, where there has been pressure put on the connective tissue while carrying the baby. All women have a belly for the first four to eight weeks after birth until the uterus shrinks back to size, but for some, the shelf can last for months or years.

Endermologie®

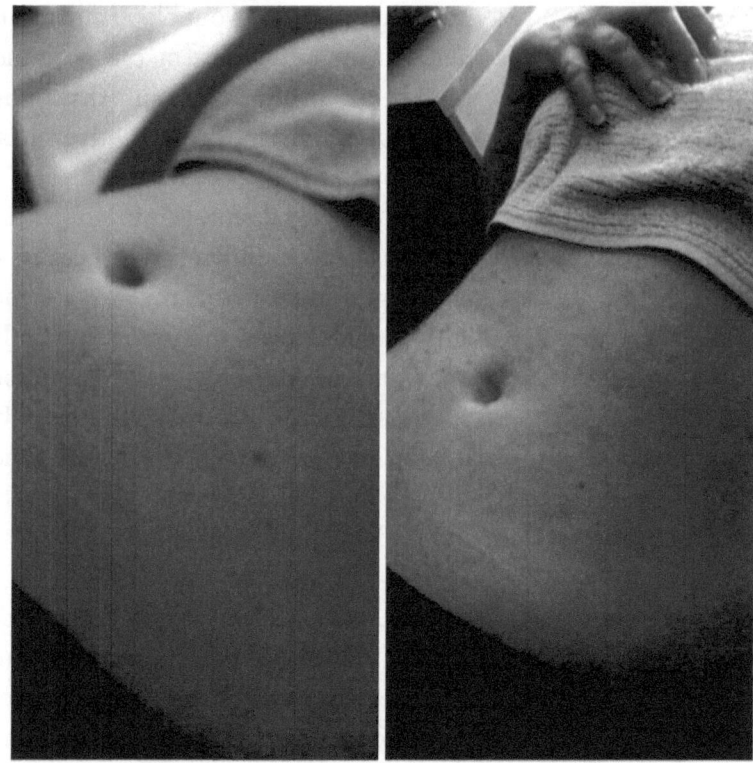

Gut issues reduced in one treatment

Breastfeeding can tighten the belly to an extent, as it causes the uterus to contract quickly and shrink. However, breastfeeding sometimes is not possible for all women. Endermologie® can break post baby fat up and tighten all the loose skin. The ab muscles called the rectus abdominis or your six pack muscles, actually separate down the front of your gut during pregnancy to make room for the baby. This can also cause issues and cause fatty deposits to form in areas you never had before.

Endermologie® rollers can get into these areas and help heal the damaged tissue to unblock and get that smooth flat tummy.

In men, their main concern is a fat gut that can cause back pain, less flexibility getting in and out of trucks and vehicles. Sit-ups sometimes are so painful and can't shift the blockages that have formed from years of beer and takeaway food. I have learnt never to say to a man he can't have his beer; it's like cutting his hand off. So, we compromise and reduce back on the alcohol and swap some foods and results start happening.

I believe it's essential for men to have that social part of a few drinks with their mates at the pub to let go of stress in the Aussie spirit. We have a local pub, golf club and workers club in town where people will come up and have a chat with you, tell a good joke, slap on the back and stumble home...occasionally stopping to lean too hard on our letterboxes. This is a town joke! You may not understand it if you're not from here.

Lymphatic Drainage

Lymphatic drainage is the most critical part of endermologie®. If we don't drain away from the toxins out of the fat cells, it just stays in the body and congests up because the body is lazy. I always drain the lymph nodes, as I love the feeling when you feel the sticky, gunk moving through, especially from the armpits that are like rubbish bins that don't get emptied or the groin area to drain and flush the ovaries and prostate.

It's so important to drain our nodes and lymph system, so there is no back-log up in our systems that create lumps and bumps that shouldn't be in our body. Blockages or fat lumps are a daily occurrence for me doing endermologie® on clients, as our lymph system only works in one direction. The lymph system doesn't have a pump like the heart that pumps the blood along, so it can get lazy as it needs the muscles to move it.

Lumps are not always fatty deposits; you can form the nasty ones too when your body becomes blocked, toxic and you don't change your lifestyle. Endermologie® helps prevent these from forming by flushing your lymph system out, and the great news is you possibly will lose a kilo a week if you follow the endermologie® weight-loss protocol with it. Included in this protocol is an easy to follow food swaps, so you never have to diet again...it's easy peasy! Over the years, numerous times I have found lumps where I stop the treatment, that the client didn't even know they had and thanks to endermologie® they were able to save their lives by acting quickly with their GP. The follow up protocol prevented more from forming and helped flush the body of the cause of the lumps.

Food Swaps

As a Nutritionist, I did years of study, doing meal plans up for different issues or health concerns and over these years I realised there was a pattern happening, clients could not stick to the meal plans, it was all too hard. I then learnt how easy it is to swap foods and eat healthily, so I designed a simple food plan of just ***swapping foods***. You must eat food from all the food groups. This can be prevented, if your family for generations has copied eating the same foods. Your great grandmother passed recipes onto her mother, and so on. Eating the same foods or lack of other food groups can cause problems or disease in the body and change your DNA. If we can change the nutrition, your DNA can alter your genes, and you can finally feel your health improve.

The reason is before we swap some foods we need toxins to be detoxed out of the body, so they don't hold your energy back or cause a foggy brain, lack of motivation and concentration.

I usually find after about 1-4 treatments, endermologie® kicks in, and you get the 'wow factor' feeling, with the body also responding to all the detoxing and food swaps. Suddenly, the inches are dropping off in areas that they have never before been able to; body pain reduces, increased flexibility and being able to move quicker.

Weight-Loss and Cellulite

One client was in so much pain with her feet, could hardly walk by the end of the day, and she needed to be on her feet for work the whole day. After five treatments, her whole demeanour changed, the pain was gone, and she could enjoy her job and her life. I love it! When clients bounce in to get their next treatment energised, instead of dragging their feet as in the first treatment. I always get the comment 'I can't wait to have Charlie'.

You don't have to eat less; you just have to eat right.
Apexathleticapparel.com

CHAPTER 2
Anxiety and Depression

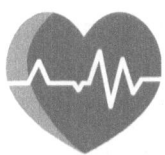

> Living with anxiety is like being followed by a voice. It knows all your insecurities and uses them against you. It gets to the point when it's the loudest voice in the room. The only one you can hear.
>
> -Healthyplace.com

Are you that person that is in a stressful job that is carrying a load of anxiety or weighing the world heavily on your shoulders with depression?

Is the stress from being away from the family, FIFO, or high expectations at work such as in the mines with the long hours as a shift-worker affecting you?

The social media and society can bombard us with messages of needing to be more, and that's one of the big reasons anxiety and depression are so prevalent. We are working so much more these days, and we are so much busier, we never get to stop and rest and rejuvenate.

Lack of nutrition, the foods we eat, fluids we drink, drugs, medications, environmental toxins, stressful situations, smoking and alcohol can all set off our anxiety, especially if consumed before the age of 16 – 18 years. These are components that can alter our DNA and cause anxiety and depression. Allowing a child to drink alcohol before 16 years can possibly turn on the alcoholic genes or smoking pot at an early age can possibly turn on the anxiety, depression and Bipolar genes later on in life. Getting your teenager through those experimental years… good luck! without alcohol and drugs, sets up their foundation for good mental health. Even if it's genetics; your great grandmother, grandmother, mother, up to three generations back passes down the same recipes, you eat similar foods that can cause your genes to change to cause anxiety and depression.

I have had clients come to me and completely get rid of all anxiety and depression after swapping foods, detoxing toxic hormones, reducing histamine levels, putting down the groundwork for a healthy DNA, reducing stress and improving their lifestyles.

It is so essential to deal with mental health issues now. Don't let this go on in your life as you may get to a point when you get too far down the path. I frequently have clients that have left it too long and are on the verge of a mental breakdown, especially when we are in the middle of a pandemic. This COVID pandemic has done massive damage to our mental health in our communities and country.

Being in lock-down, not being able to connect with our families or friends and feeling so isolated has caused people to become anxious, depressed, worried and angry at being told what to do. Even as our country heals, we now have the after effects of COVID with our mental health.

Anxiety and Depression

Why is stress, anxiety, depression and mental health issues becoming so common? One cause is a detoxing issue in the brain. When we go to sleep, our brain gets detoxed but if you're not getting your 7.5 hours of uninterrupted sleep you are possibly not allowing the body to do its natural course of detoxing when you sleep. Clients that have had sleep issues improved feel calmer.

I often get so many clients that have Anxiety, Depression, PTSD, come to see me on antidepressants and medication saying, it's just not working, or they are putting on so much weight. This is where their lifestyles need to be changed and extra help is required while still taking medication.

Cerebrospinal Fluid

Did you know the brain's cerebrospinal fluid (CSF) pulses during your sleep and helps to flush out toxic memory-impairing proteins from the brain?

This process can get blocked, and often clients will have tense or sore neck and shoulders. This instantly tells me, not enough blood flow is getting to the brain. The lymph system flows in one direction... up and dumps in the upper part of the body into the bloodstream. This can get blocked and accumulate, not allowing the natural process of CSF pulses to flush.

The endermologie® protocol I designed for anxiety and depression rolls up and down the spine flushing this CSF and clearing out blocked lymph, especially the hump behind the neck that forms and possibly can help flush toxic memory-impairing proteins from the brain.

When the neurotransmitters or our chemicals in the brain don't work correctly and have malfunctions or imbalance, they can cause effects such as mood swings, anger, anxiety and depression. It becomes unbalanced through our lifestyles of inadequate nutrition, stress, alcohol, drugs and environmental toxins. Understanding which neurotransmitter and how it is unbalanced is essential.

Let me explain the brain chemicals, so you have a clear understanding of what is happening to you. Stay with me, it may get a bit complicated, but it's so important for you to understand what is going on in your head.

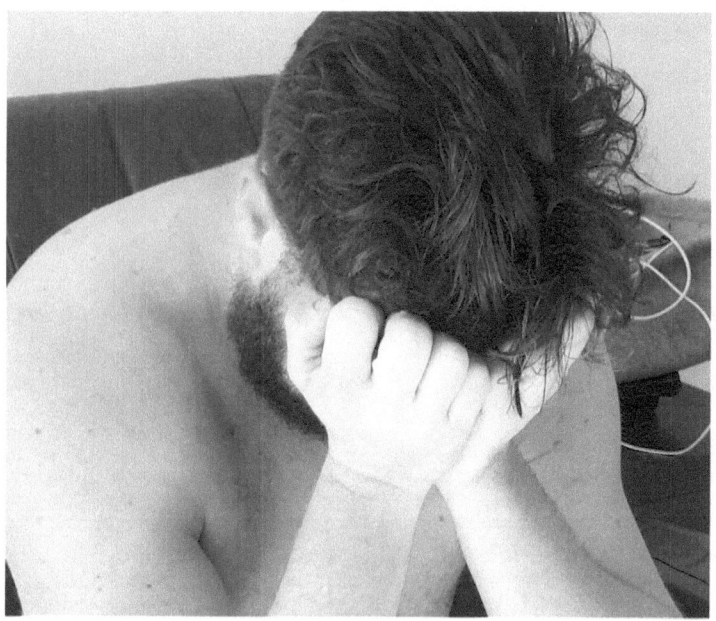

Seven Neurotransmitters

The seven neurotransmitters in the brain are glutamate, gamma-aminobutyric acid (GABBA), acetylcholine, dopamine, histamine, norepinephrine and serotonin. I am a DNA analyst and enjoy working so much on the client's genes, as they hold so many answers to their unbalanced chemicals in the brain and health issues. Here is a list of the seven neurotransmitters;

Glutamate that excites and sends signals to the nerve cells and is vital in learning and memory.

GABBA is very important as it reduces and controls the fear or anxiety when the brain cells are over-excited. Altered levels in GABBA can cause depression, anxiety and neurodegenerative diseases like Alzheimer's and ageing.

Acetylcholine activates the muscles, and too much can cause cramps, increased salivation, muscular weakness, blurry vision, diarrhoea, slow heart rate, dilated blood vessels, to name a few. Sorry to my caffeine-addicted clients, but caffeine can also increase acetylcholine, causing these symptoms. Too little acetylcholine can cause Alzheimer's, Parkinson's disease, muscle weakness, memory loss, depression and anxiety and this is why it is so important to have a balance.

Dopamine is a feel-good, happy neurotransmitter and is released with pleasurable situations such as food, coffee, sex, drugs and alcohol. Too little can lead to Parkinson's but too high can lead to high libido, anxiety, sleep issues, increased energy, addictive behaviours, mania, hallucinations, PTSD and schizophrenia. Stress reduces dopamine.

Understanding smoking and the effects on our neurotransmitters are important, as nicotine is sent to the brain and attaches to the nicotine receptors. It releases dopamine, and that's why you feel good when you smoke but also causes an imbalance of dopamine and this is one of the reasons it is tough to give up smoking. Alcohol also causes a dopamine release that feels great when you are drinking, but 3-4 days later can cause unexplained mood swings such as anger, frustration and depression. Alcohol is similar to a depressant as when you drink it, you become relaxed, yet so many people drink because they are depressed.

Histamine promotes wakefulness. With a histamine disorder, you can experience brain fog, sinus issues, inflammation in the body, skin issues, headaches, migraines, fatigue, irregular menstrual cycle, skin issues and anxiety. It relates to all the smooth muscle in the body such as tissues in the lungs, uterus and gut causing lowered blood pressure, hormonal issues and water weight.

Norepinephrine increases arousal, alertness, energy, attention, emotions, sleeping, dreaming and learning. Having too much norepinephrine or adrenaline can cause high blood pressure, excessive sweating, anxiety, panic attacks and hyperactivity. Not enough norepinephrine can cause attention deficit hyperactivity disorder (ADHD) and depression.

Finally, **Serotonin** is the one to feel-good, positive feelings, pleasure and love. It regulates happiness, PTSD, depression and anxiety. Caffeine, alcohol and nicotine can decrease serotonin, and serotonin is a precursor to melatonin that helps you sleep.

I also want to mention one more **Substance p** is for the transmission of pain, information found in the brain and spinal cord and an imbalance can make you uncomfortable, in pain, wired energy with skin sensations. It is three times higher in fibromyalgia, CSF leak and PTSD. Endermologie® can also help to improve Fibromyalgia and remember, we also want to enhance the CSF to improve anxiety and depression, all related to the neurotransmitters in the brain.

As stated before, all these neurotransmitters can become unbalanced by drugs, alcohol, smoking, lack of good nutrition, environmental toxins such as high mercury that can lead to Dementia and a big issue is self-supplementation.

Dr Joseph Pizzorno studies show diseases associated with our environmental toxins:
Arsenic - cancers, diabetes, gout
DDT (sprayed in our streets in the 60s) - ADHD, dementia, diabetes
Phthalates - ADHD, diabetes
PBDEs - ADHD, diabetes
PHAs - ADHD, cancers, MI, RA
Mercury - Dementia
Lead – Cardiovascular disease, IQ (2018 Pizzorno, Dr J)

The internet is flooding us with information on how supplements can do so many benefits, but there are hidden ingredients that increase the neurotransmitters that can unbalance the brain chemicals. I had a client come in to see me feeling as if she was losing her mind with manic tendencies. After a naturopathic consultation, I was able to find out the cause of the supplement she was taking and then detox it out of her tissue to calm her back down. Her husband was very appreciative.

Endermologie® can bring you back to the start, by eliminating toxins, possibly the cause of the fluctuations in your neurotransmitters. We need to teach the body to flush itself, getting the body to create new fresh, healthy brain cells with detoxing and using the CSF protocol.

There is good news; we are still able to produce new brain cells with neurogenesis, a process of generating new neurons in the brain. The cells that are in the hippocampus tend to shrink as we get heavy metal toxicity, ageing, lack of nutrition, to name a few, and we get loss of learning. These changes to the hippocampus can reverse by creating new cells. A study showed that exercise increases and produces new cells in the brain and improves learning and cognitive improvement. It also found that running has the same effect as an antidepressant due to a drop in the stress hormones. (2003 Tomporowski Phillip) When exercising, blood flow is increased, and endermologie® can create the same process. It increases the blood flow by 400% and using exercise as well; your body will reach huge healthy levels. I always encourage a 1km shuffle jog per day. It's a slow jog just a little faster than a walk, where you can talk to the person next to you without getting out of breath, still getting your heart pumping and putting no stress on your body. The results are excellent!

The protocol I use for mental health stress is, the machine rolls up the spine using different moves with the endermologie® head and promotes blood flow into the brain. Within minutes of blood flow being stimulated up the spine, the client instantly releases all tension and stress. It's like having a detox session to the brain and helps you to sleep better, with often clients falling asleep in the hour session. Any treatment that allows you to sleep better is going to help the CSF work its magic while you sleep and also to help you wake up in the morning and leap out of bed happy and revitalised. Who doesn't want that! With the combination of 'calm the farm' herbal tonic, supplements, testing your DNA to balance brain chemicals and understanding the genes that are affecting you, is a must.

Hope that wasn't too much information for you but if I can simplify it for you, it can make those easy changes without having to go down that path of medication. However, I do agree with medicating, when you are at that point in your life you have left it too long, go to your GP immediately and get on medication and as I say to my clients, we can mop up later with treatments, tonics, teas and supplements and work in conjunction with your integrated GP.

> It's so difficult to describe depression to someone who's never been there because it's not sadness. I know sadness. Sadness is to cry and to feel. But it's that cold absence of feeling – that hollowed-out feeling."
> **-J.K.Rowling**

CHAPTER 3

Menopause

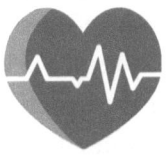

"I don't have hot flashes; I have short, private vacations in tropical-like conditions."
-Live Better With Menopause

Has your body slowed down, tired, moods just over the top, snapping at everyone and trying to deal with the hideous deliberating menopause symptoms? Living in our amazing town out in Moranbah, we absorb our environmental toxins. I love living here; the people are so awesome and my passion is to keep as many people healthy while working out here.

This is the main reason I live here, is the satisfaction in the results I get, detoxing as many people as possible and keeping them healthy and happy. As we age, our body has more difficulty ridding of environmental and hormonal toxins, especially in menopause. We take on all the toxins in our foods, water and environment, especially

Endermologie®

plastics as the plastics cause xenoestrogens or toxic estrogen in our liver that can also cause menopause symptoms on top of our body's excess hormonal oestrogen.

The endermologie® procedure for menopause goes in and flushes out the liver, kidneys and ovaries. Even if the menopause phase has kicked in and shrunk the ovaries, it's essential to flush that area. Using a rolling technique, the rollers promote excess blood flow to these areas. As well, the rollers can focus on flushing the uterus with so much blood flow, the cells possibly can renew and can promote thickening of the uterus depending on your stage in menopause. One client after five treatments, her periods came back slowing the menopause phase down. The menopause protocol includes a flush to the lymph system, the lymph nodes, under the arms and around the groin area. As the lymph moves in a one-way direction and doesn't have anything to pump it along; it relies on motions of the muscles to pump, and then it dumps into the bloodstream but if we sit at a desk all day, this blocks the lymph up. This is why we have to exercise with menopause; we have to move. Exercising in the morning is always the best as it gets the body moving and sets you up for the day.

After the endermologie® menopause protocol, the lymph system is flushed so much that often the next day the bowels can excrete excess mucus. Toxins can accumulate in the body due to these blocked lymph nodes. Breaking the lymph gunk up is so satisfying and feeling that gunk shift through. I also encourage a teaspoon of apple cider vinegar in a mug of warm water in the morning as the potassium content is excellent to break up the mucus in the lymph as we aren't exercising, sitting down a lot during the day like most of my truck drivers, we can become stagnant.

This menopause protocol I use completes two treatments in one session, especially on the gut as this is another main area that blocks up. The liver can get so blocked with toxins, it has nowhere to put them. The toxins will get stored in the fat cells around the gut to protect the toxicity from entering the bloodstream. Our body is incredible with all the processes and pathways that go to work to protect the body. The first 30 minute treatment breaks it down and flushes away, then the next 30 minute treatment does the same, but it goes deeper into the next layer like an onion peeling back layer after layer. Following is the infra-red-ray wrap (the straps wrap) I also use where the fat cells are again flushed. This can cause a reduction in the fat cells around the gut as the toxins are flushed out twice and is really noticeable over the next 3 days through the bowels or kidneys.

Sorry to burst your bubble but fat cells don't disappear. We need them, but they can reduce in size. They are white fat cells or adipose tissue, and they can shrink, and this is what endermologie® process possibly can help to achieve by shrinking your fat cells. The sad news is, your fat cells will expand again quickly due to your lifestyle habits that caused it in the first place. This is why you put weight back on quickly, especially in menopause. Learning the food swaps and changing the way you live is not tricky. The great news is the endermologie® teaches the body to drain and flush the fat cells, causing belly fat to shrink that forms during menopause. Regular weekly or fortnightly treatments are required till all your symptoms have gone.

Then maintenance of once a month will be needed. Quite often, clients will come back and say I feel I have come down 1-2 dress sizes, but I'm still the same weight. Endermologie® can promote the body to shrink and crack the fat cells while sculpting the body of areas that are difficult to move. The weight is due to the amount of food you eat. This process can become easy with endermologie®, as the machine motivates you to get moving and promotes better eating. As you feel so good, you aren't turning to comfort food anymore. Of course, we then work on the nutrition aspect of swapping foods around. Remember NO dieting that's no fun, just food swaps. I don't even like to use the word diet. It has the word 'die' in it and immediately associates pain with it. We all need to learn to eat from all food groups with a balanced food plan that gives the body a wide range of vitamins, minerals, fats, proteins and carbohydrates. Food is energy, and it is the best supplementation for the body.

Menopause Phase

During the menopause phase, the ovaries don't produce estrogen anymore and slowly shrink down, but the estrogen can still be made by other parts of the body. The adrenal glands and the fat tissue can take over producing estrogen, and even studies have shown that the brain can produce estrogen. The research indicates that the hypothalamus in the brain is capable of making estrogen and that it may also act as a neurotransmitter in the brain. (2014 Barcley, Rachel)

So, you ask yourself why is there menopause if other parts of our body take over and produce estrogen? It is simple, our bodies get blocked with our environmental toxins we take on over our lifetime, and our organs in our body are exhausted, especially the adrenals from being too busy all the time. Being 'busy' all the time is the new emotion of not having enough time to spend on yourself. It is therefore important not to wear our adrenals out because these are our back up for menopause. How brilliant is our body to organise the adrenals and fat tissue to take over from the ovaries and produce our estrogen? If this process is happening, then we ought not to have menopause symptoms or hot flushes and mood swings.

Plastics

Stay with me; we need to understand plastics as well, how it can affect menopause and the health of our body. We drink from plastic bottles; food is packaged in plastic, and we even freeze in plastic. BPA is a synthetic estrogen found in many plastic products, food, formulas, can linings, dental sealants, cashier receipts used to stabilise the ink. BPA is a hormone disruptor that can cause obesity, infertility and hormonal issues such as menopause. A lot of us are not aware that even though your bottle is BPA free, it can be substituted with BPF and BPS that is still bisphenol and has the same toxic levels as BPA.

The heat from washing the containers with Bisphenols A,B or S can release toxins into our foods and water. A study was done on washing plastic bottles in hot water after use and the environmental toxin estrogen, BPA was released 55 times more rapidly. This BPA is an endocrine disruptor and can alter the body by mimicking the role of your hormones. All used in reusable water bottles, food linings, water pipes and dental sealants, to name a few. (2008 University of Cincinnati)

Environmental Plastics

Here are plastics broken down for you into their categories;

#1 Polyethylene Terephthalate (PET, PETE, Polyester) used in bottled water, juice, salad dressings, microwavable food trays. It can be used once, but it's porous and collects germs and toxins so leaving a bottle in the car heats it and leeches the toxins.

#2 High-Density Polyethylene (HDPE) found in milk cartons, detergents, plastic bags, freezer bags.

#3 Polyvinyl Chloride (PVC) Is plastic in many products and phthalates are added to the PVC. It is in our shampoo, nail polish, hair spray. It can cause endocrine disruption with reduced sperm count and liver cancer.

#4 Low-Density Polyethylene (LDPE) found in plastic bags, food storage containers, squeezable bottles

#5 Polypropylene (PP) This is a thicker plastic found in yoghurt, margarine, bottle caps, food storage containers, some water filters, storage bins, diapers/sanitary pads.

#6 Polystyrene (PS) is used for meat trays, food containers it leaches hormone disruptors.

> #7 Other plastics have BPA in it and can cause cancer, obesity, endocrine disruption. (2016 Schwartz, Larry)

Let's use a glass!

Endermologie® can promote the body to flush out the liver of these plastic xenoestrogens, out of the tissue to stimulate healthy cells. I love to follow up with my detoxing herbs such as *Taraxacum officinale Cynara scolymus* or many other herbal remedies to suit the individual. My favourite supplements are Indol Carbonol 3 or DIM. These are very powerful to get toxic oestrogen out of the liver, but there is a unique protocol to follow on how to take them, so please check with your health practitioner.

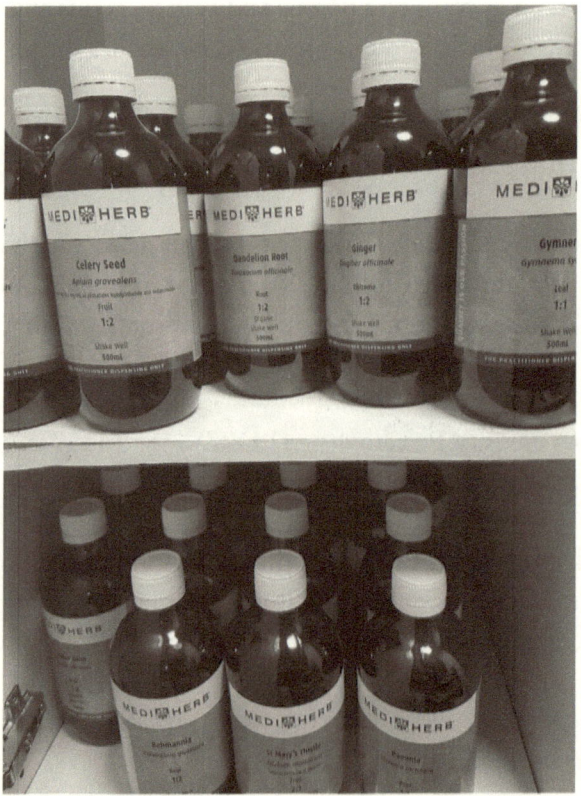

Estrogen Pathways

As stated before, environmental xenoestrogens/hormonal oestrogens are stored in our liver and tissue and over the years they can build up in the body and cause all sorts of health issues such as; breast, cervical, and prostate cancer and possibly miscarriages.

Oestrogen is metabolised through the liver in three pathways and depending on the pathway used; the oestrogen will be converted into good or bad metabolites. The pathway called 2-hydroxy is good; the 16-hydroxy and 4-hydroxy paths are the ones associated with cancer, especially breast cancer. So, it makes sense if you have the breast cancer genes to learn to keep these pathways cleared.

As explained by Preston, when your body uses the 2-hydroxy pathway, you will produce good estrogen that gives you a healthy mood, libido, fertility and healthy breast tissue. Now if your body gets overloaded or blocked with plastics and environmental toxins or converting too many hormones, it will use the 4-hydroxy and 16-hydroxy pathways, and this is bad. It's called oestrogen dominance, and this is where at an early age, you can get PMS, irritability, heavy periods to name a few. Then if you carry later on in life without making health changes and don't detox, symptoms of vaginal dryness, hot flushes, mood swings or even a high risk of getting breast cancer can occur. Then our genes get compromised, especially the major one methylenetetrahydrofolate (MTHFR) or COMT genes that can't detoxify these hormones and they continue to build in the liver. (2020 Preston ND, Cynthia) These plastics, as well as other issues of molds, parasites, yeast and candida overgrowth, can all pollute our body and can change our body health negatively.

MTHFR

Our genes get compromised, especially the major one MTHFR or related genes such as the COMT, PON1 genes that can't detoxify our environmental toxins and hormones.

Over the years, I have tested many clients' genes, and only one person has ever not had the MTHFR gene. However, once the client finds out they do have it, and the type, whether it's MTHFR C677T or A1298C heterozygous or homozygous or the compounding genes, their lives can change dramatically by understanding the protocol to use. The most difficult genes to help are the MTHFR compounding as it can feel as if you're being pulled in two different directions and I do find they are the hardest to treat.

In menopause, the COMT gene can be increased as the oestrogen levels decline. The COMT gene is important as it gives instructions for making an enzyme called catechol-O-methyltransferase. If there is a variation in this gene, it limits the body's ability to remove catechols such as excess dopamine, norepinephrine and estrogen. This causes higher levels of cortisol causing the body to find it hard to calm itself and destress. If you have issues with the COMT gene, it can affect your hormones, especially during the menopause phase, causing more neurotic behaviour and lower stress resiliency. (2020 Davis, Tchiki PhD)

Oestrogen Deficiency

There are not only issues affecting environmental oestrogens entering our body and causing cancer-related problems and menopause, but there is an estrogen deficiency. It affects our serotonin levels that can cause mood swings, depression and urinary tract infections due to the thinning of the tissue in the uterus. The endermologie® can help promote the body to flush blood flow to the liver, tissues, uterus and ovaries to help reduce all these symptoms.

You can have bloods taken to check if your body is still producing enough oestrogen, but you also know by your periods becoming less and less. I just tell my clients to; detox the toxins out with endermologie®, eat oestrogen foods, take herbal teas and tonics to produce more oestrogen, tweak your genes MTHFR and COMT and stop being busy all the time wearing your adrenals down by stressing and getting adrenal fatigue.

Adrenal fatigue is our new emotion 'I'm so busy'. We are all too busy to look after our health, to exercise, or to meditate for a calm, healthy mind. This emotion is an excuse for you not to put your health first; it's an excuse to self-sabotage your health.

Menopause Stages

The stages of menopause are, perimenopause when you have had 12 months of no period. The postmenopausal stage is when it's been 24-36 months after your last period. Estradiol is the main form of estrogen in our body, and the average level is 30-400 pg/mL, and after menopause, it can drop below 30pg/mL.

There are foods containing natural compounds that provide oestrogen effects such as soy-based products of tofu, tempeh and miso. Still, it is essential to get organic, or you are just going to put the environmental toxins back in that are causing your menopause issues. As stated by Galvin and Bishop, other plant-based foods that contain phyto-oestrogens can reduce the hot flushes, vaginal dryness and lower breast cancer risk such as; chickpeas, soybeans, split peas, mung beans, lentils, broad beans, alfalfa, flaxseed and rye. The phyto-oestrogen foods can mimic oestrogen in the body by binding to our oestrogen receptors while soy can increase bone health and prevent osteoporosis. (2011 Galvin, K. Bishop M.)

Some amazing herbs I use in conjunction with endermologie® for menopause are; *Cimicifuga racemose, Hypericum perforatum, Asparagus racemosus, Zizyphus Spinosa, Dioscorea villosa,* to name a few. Or some of my favourite calming teas are; *Salvia officinalis, Passiflora incarnata, Lavendula angustifolia.* Please remember you can't self-medicate herbs, it's important to see your practitioner for correct dosage and use as we have spent years at University studying positive and negative aspects of the herbs and the interactions with medications. Herbal plant food is healthy and can help to shift all those deliberating symptoms of menopause while your system is flushing with endermologie®. Herbs are my passion, and they are natural plant food, and I just love them.

"Not to brag or anything, but I can forget what I am doing, while I am doing it."
-Live Better With Menopause

CHAPTER 4

Children

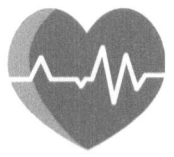

'Children learn more from what you are than what you teach.'

-W.E.B. DuBois

Is your child stressing or full of anxiety? Hates going to school? Or continually getting into trouble at school? Or having constant gut pain? Toxicity of heavy metals in children is common, and we don't even realise it. Toxicity can be from their environment or even passed on in the womb. Treating children with endermologie® is so much fun and satisfying. The kids just adore endermologie®, and as soon as I run the rollers down their backs and promote blood flow to the nervous system, they instantly relax. I use smaller rollers on them depending on their fat, age and muscle content.

The younger kids usually need a hand by mum getting into the endermowear™, as they often end up in a tangle first go. But once they know how to put it on, there is usually a race to get into it and lie down on the treatment table. I get such satisfaction treating children as they respond so quickly. After a treatment, most will go home and sleep deeply while the body detoxes.

I always encourage everyone to drink water to flush out the toxins and to bring a water bottle to their treatment, so as soon as they sit up, the flushing process starts and also to train them to always have a water bottle on them . I love the positive feedback from their parents about what the teachers say, how they have settled in class with improved concentration. I still remember one feedback I got from a ten-year old boy; how he could run faster and he doesn't get angry anymore. I had tears in my eyes as I just feel so passionate about making a 100% change in a child, the positive changes in the way they feel emotionally and how they react to stressful situations.

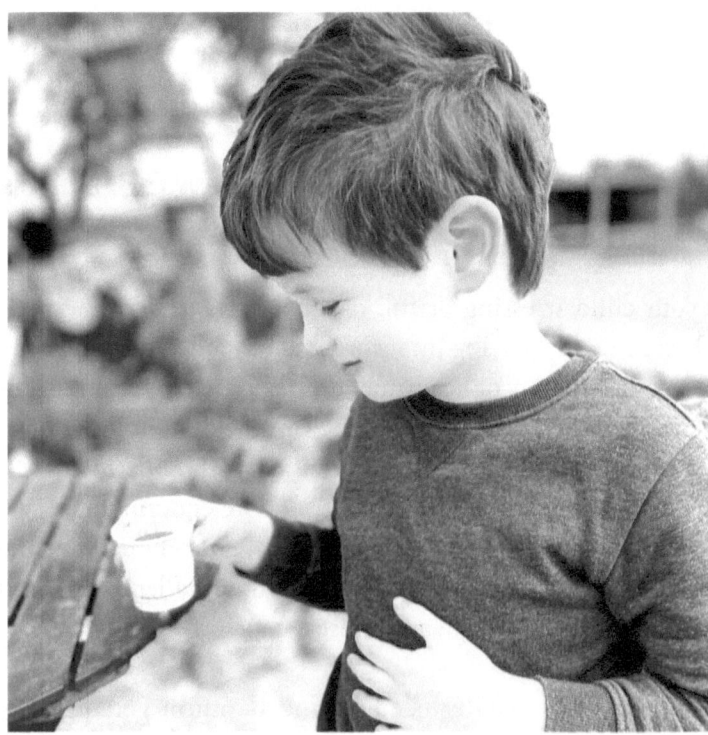

Growth Plates

Growth plates are areas of new bone growth that consist of cartilage. The growth plates are usually situated near the long bones. A girl's growth plates will close when they are approximately 14-15 years old while boys will close around 16-17 years, but it can depend on the child as well and can close at different times. (2020 Kuester Dr Victoria) These growth plates can give a child so much pain they can get to a stage of having issues walking and playing sport. The endermologie® procedure can help growth plate issues in a child.

For the child, the endermologie® treatment I use first starts by running down the back as this helps to relax the nervous system and they instantly sigh, and I can see their eyes begin to close within minutes. The size of the head I use depends on the age. The rollers also run down the legs and buttocks releasing lactic acid and promoting healthy blood flow. Children will get growing pains or even severe pain from their growth plates, but endermologie® can promote healing very fast.

I also enjoy treating Calcaneal Apophysitis that is a painful inflammation of the heel's growth plate. It usually affects children 8-14 years of age. Included in the protocol is the foot, releasing of the Achilles heel and up into the calf muscle. There can be instant relief with endermologie® and their injuries, and releasing the acid from their joints to prevent future injuries.

Injuries on children are rapid to heal with endermologie®. I had a child with an injury to his collarbone. We focused on flushing out the inflammation on the area, and the next morning he woke up with hardly any pain. Children react and improve nearly instantly with endermologie®. However, the biggest challenge is to keep them still with an injury and allow it time to heal.

The endermologie® treatment programme for the children is for the age group of 7-16 years. I not only focus on treating their lymph glands and lymph nodes but also the gut. I treat a lot of children with Functional Abdominal Pain (FAP) that is very painful in the stomach and can be very disturbing for the child, possibly due to stress and anxiety. If the gut has pain, there are also gut lining problems, and this can prevent absorbing vital minerals and vitamins needed to keep their energy and brain health at an optimal level.

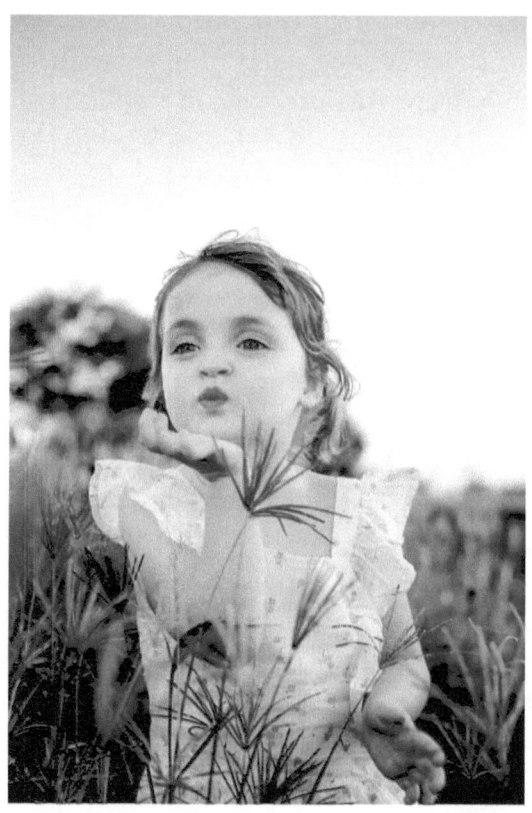

Gently running the rollers over the gut area can be similar to a gentle cleansing process of the gut that promotes the blood flow to come in and flush it out. Often the bowels can get released, and the child will have a healthy clean out and feel pain-free.

Flushing the bowels is important as it's like putting the rubbish bin out; it's our dumping ground, and we need to keep it working at an optimal level. A child that doesn't poop daily is cranky with low mood and energy levels. We need to promote blood flow and oxygenation to all the major organs.

Minerals

One of the significant problems I get here in town is an imbalance of minerals, especially iron with children. We are in a coal mine town, so their little body gets blocked and can't absorb.

Absorbing minerals in the body are like having car parks. If toxins enter the body, then they take over the car parks where the minerals are meant to be, and even if you take supplements, the body may not be able to absorb them due to the heavy metals taking over the carparks and not allowing the minerals back in—a bit like carpark road rage.

The endermologie® protocol can come in and kick the toxins out of the mineral carparks, increase blood flow and helps the body to oxygenate and start absorbing their beautiful minerals and vitamins. Then, foods high in iron can be absorbed or possibly an iron supplement helps to re-balance the minerals out again. If bloods have been taken, we can then supplement, as we don't ever supplement iron without bloodwork, as an overload of iron can make your child very sick.

Never, ever self-supplement your child with iron without a blood test or hair mineral test as this can cause serious health issues. The hair mineral test report I do is fantastic but it took me over 2 years of study to learn the ratios of all the minerals and the effects, especially related to living in a coal mine town. If you do your own hair mineral test, it's important to go to a qualified practitioner as the report doesn't explain how to treat the cross over ratios of the minerals that are very important.

Anemia is so common in children when there is a lack of iron out here in the mines. Anemia can be the lack of oxygen-carrying the red blood cells. However too much iron in the body can cause aggressive behaviour, hyperactivity and too little iron can affect children's neuronal development in the brain or infections in the body. It's essential to learn why the body is not utilising or absorbing iron. 'The body can utilise iron only if the stomach has an acidic environment. A lack of normal acidity in the stomach will reduce iron absorption in the small intestine.' (2010 Dr David L Watts)

This acid environment in the gut has digestive enzymes, and hydrochloric acid is needed to break the food down to absorb the iron. Some foods neutralise these acids, and some foods increase the acid in the gut, such as fermented foods. Now if your child has issues with their Histamine genes, then these fermented foods are going to cause more health issues. This is going to start the problems with the skin, eczema, dermatitis, sinusitis, and even anxiety. This is an example of only one mineral.

Treating children out in the mines is my favourite area with their minerals and their imbalance. Another example, is too much copper from our copper pipes still used in the older style homes, can also cause a lack of iron and even depression.

Doing an endermologie® treatment on a child first helps to flush out the toxins that are taking up the minerals carparks before we supplement. Often the blood tests reflect the iron supplement isn't working, or it's storing in the tissue and not being absorbed. Remove the toxin and balance the acid out in the gut with endermologie® to help balance out their minerals by reducing the heavy metal load.

Another area effecting iron absorption is oxalates. Your practitioner can look at your heavy load of food oxalates in the body or possibly your DNA oxalate genes to determine whether the oxalates are also inhibiting iron absorption by combining with the iron to form iron oxide and that's bad. There are many components to looking at mineral imbalances and understanding the cross-over ratios.

Children

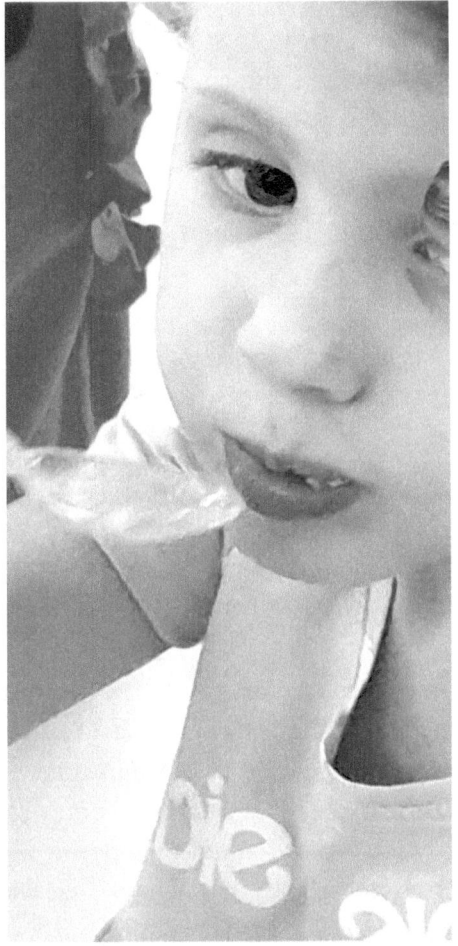

Over supplementing or self-medicating kids is very common in parents these days. They are consumed with the internet and Facebook advertising and all these supplements and products that contain herbs, oils and ingredients that can be very dangerous for children's mental health and digestive systems to absorb. I constantly see children that are being poisoned by over use of supplements. For example, taking a simple magnesium supplement without realising there are poorly absorbed ones, inorganic, or the types of magnesium for totally different reasons for the body.

> Magnesium Threonate can cross the brain barrier and is great for the nervous system and memory, but too much can start to change our DNA, possibly affecting their brain chemicals.

> Magnesium Citrate is great for leg cramps and helps promote sleep, but it's not advisable with high histamine issues that cause anxiety.

> Magnesium Malate that is energising and produces ATP that is energy in our body, but suddenly parents are tearing their hair out when the child is tearing around over energised.

> Magnesium Glycinate does the opposite and calms the body but is not advised in high oxalate people because it possibly causes issues with thyroid and joints.

The other big problem poor parents face is fussy eaters. I had one of those with my daughter growing up and I feel for those parents. Every night for sixteen years I went through this with my daughter saying 'I don't like that' every time her meat and vegetables were put in front of her. My son was the complete opposite. He ate everything and absolutely loved food. With these fussy eaters we find, once they have had endermologie® the toxins are coming out of their little bodies and there is less cravings for comfort foods of sugar and takeaway. Teaching the parents how to become smart in hiding vegetables in other foods and endermologie® treatments regularly to keep the environmental toxins out, is the missing link to a healthier mind and body in our children.

Growth Stretch Marks

Stretch marks are another treatment I do for many teenagers. Stretch marks are common with puberty in girls and boys when they are growing quickly. Usually in girls on the breasts, buttocks and legs. The endermologie® was first designed in the 1980's to treat burn and scar victims with the amazing technology, with the rollers promoting collagen and elastin in the skin to heal very quickly. It is one of the world's number one treatments for the skin. The stretch marks can possibly completely go away if they are still coloured but if they have been left too long and turn white, we can then smooth the scar and make it look less visible. So, it's important to get onto them straight away. How long treating with endermologie® depends on the child's body growth and healing of their skin; but usually eight to ten treatments.

Anxiety

I see a lot of children with anxiety out here and it's possibly due to the environmental toxins but also our kids these days are so busy. When they finish school, they are off to their sports groups that are so important to learn teamwork. Sometimes their days can be really long and very hot. I have some very gentle anxiety and low mood tonics for children that can 'calm the farm,' nourish the neurotransmitters, reduce their stress levels so they are able to cope with everyday activities at school and home.

If we look at the statistics, anxiety is increasing everywhere for children. The Australian Government statistics says; anxiety disorders are the second most common disorder at 6.9% and among girls it's 6.1%. In 2013 314,000 children aged 4-11 experienced a mental disorder. Boys were affected more than girls while Attention Deficit Hyperactivity Disorder, ADHD is the most common at 8.2% with boys being the highest at 11%. (2020 Australian Institute of Health and Welfare)

Mental health problems in childhood can have a substantial impact on wellbeing. There is strong evidence that mental disorders in childhood and adolescence predict mental illness in adulthood. (2020

Australian Institute of Health and Welfare) Kids get up-tight and agitated in everyday living of environmental toxins and leading such busy lifestyles. Encourage your child to attend yoga, meditation, or listen to the sound bowls to help relax and promote a healthy mind. Also, the endermologie® procedure using the rollers runs gently up the side of the spine to promote blood flow to the brain that flushes the toxins. The child is instantly less stressed and will have an amazing deep restful sleep straight after their first treatment. This promotes less stress, less anxiety and is the missing link to a happy child.

> 'Children are not things to be moulded, but are people to be unfolded'
>
> **-Jess Lair**

CHAPTER 5

Men's Health

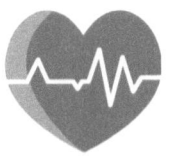

"He who cures a disease may be the skillfullest, but he that prevents it is the safest physician."
-Thomas Fuller

How frustrated are you with your man not looking after their health? Do you constantly nag them to stop drinking all the time, you know they are getting that delicious burger from the servo in Moranbah on top of their lunch you make for them? Are they silly enough to leave their takeaway rubbish in their trucks? These are stories I always hear from the partners that make me roar with laughter.

I must say those burgers out at the servo are delicious out here in Moranbah, where you can still get an original burger like back in the old days. But guys, not every day! Loaded with fries, tomato sauce and even worse, loaded up with salt. You know you can practically feel your heart squeezing with shock and your inner health child says, "that's my last one", but you're back there the very next day! You might be saying what is wrong with me that I have no self-control?

Well, I'm here to help you. It's called comfort eating and it's a cycle called self-medicating with takeaway food to feel good. Another cycle is not exercising …I'm too busy. It's an excuse you use to not look after your health. You are telling yourself I'm not worthy to look after my health because I'm putting my family, girlfriend or mates first to show how successful I am. Well, I'm here to let you know, it's all a story you're making up in your head and I have the secret to getting you out of your own head and into a healthy body.

It doesn't mean you can't go to the pub for a beer with your mates or have a barbie. It's called moderation and having a balance, so that your body can recover and keep giving you that amazing energy and deep sleep that puts you on top of the world. Your testosterone is going to increase, your energy is going to get you leaping out of bed, you will enjoy going to work, and people won't frustrate you as much anymore. How can they when you are a positive vibrant man to be around. No one wants to be around a grumpy, depressed, negative man. Let me give you the secret to help you to break free of your health issues.

Gut Issues

Your gut issues can cause bloating even if you are training hard at that gym. It can have two areas of bloating; one part is above the belly button and usually affects you, when you have just eaten that can give you warning signs, that certain foods are reacting. The other area is below the belly button and that can give you a sign that your digestive system is not working. Some men can even have both areas and it's turned into a barrel. This is dangerous and it really can put a strain on your heart with lack of blood flow to the heart. Also, you don't feel good, you're sluggish, you move slowly and you won't be getting a sound sleep because you will be snoring so loudly and your partner won't be impressed. It's a frustrating spot to be in, because to exercise it hurts and then if you do exercise often, you are putting all this hard work in and not getting results. It's like getting on a merry-go-round, you need to stop the junk food and drink less alcohol to feel better but then you don't have the energy to exercise and it makes you feel fatigued, so then you go eat and drink badly again to feel better.

Endermologie® is the missing link to bring your stomach down, shift that weight, get rid of heavy metal toxicity and to stop waking up tired in the morning and even possibly put you in a good mood. Endermologie® can help you feel amazing by bringing back your vitality, increasing your energy, balancing out your moods, and help you get off that merry-go-round of bad eating and no exercise.

As soon as my male clients arrive, I can see the blockages in the gut. It's tight, they find they don't have the flexibility to lean over. They are actually squashing their organs, when they do. This fat is called visceral fat. It develops overtime around the centre of the body and can be hard to lose once you have it. Endermologie® protocol makes it a breeze. The men definitely need the one-hour treatment when treating the gut. The first 30 minute treatment, the inflammation reduces and then the next 30 minutes I find the gut has softened, I can really get stuck into the layers and is also easier to work with when it's softer. The results are really evident instantly and I can see it reduced in size as it becomes softer and pliable. That's the trick of endermologie®. It gets into the digestive system and flushes it and the blockages are released, the gut then becomes softer and reduces in size. Often foods in the past that men have had a reaction to will cease. Heartburn and indigestion will balance as the digestion system balances and helps the gut corrects itself internally with the client following the food swap protocol as well. Many clients often come to me to see what foods are reacting but in fact the gut needs to be healed first.

Mental Health

Mental health is a huge issue out here in the mines. It's long hours and it's a toxic environment but on the positive side, it's earning an income for you to set your family up or yourself for future security. My goal is to help as many people live here in healthy states so they feel good and don't go into the funk that is so common.

Some tips are; a hobby is a great way to release stress or focus on something you enjoy. I have clients that start up having fish, teaching themselves guitar, another one runs or bike rides. Another tip is to make time with your mates, girl talk can be exhausting but just sitting with your mates and having a yarn is amazing therapy, or even organising a boys fishing trip away. Getting the rubbish out of your head that can repeat itself over and over by laughing is another great tip and the best medicine. I have to tell some men to fake two laughs a day, until it becomes a habit and it is contagious. Most important tip is water to stay hydrated and keep your minerals in-take up as it is so hot out here, you drink that much water from sweating and you can also lose your minerals. I use a combination of good quality minerals to put in your water that really boost.

If you are foggy, fatigued, cranky and snappy, it's the first sign your body is letting you know your mental health is being compromised. I know you don't want to snap at the kids or your wife or girlfriend but you can't control it. Or you're sitting in the carpark and the jealous monkey brain takes over and by the time your wife arrives back to the car, you start an argument over nothing!

It's so confusing for you and you want to stop yourself but sometimes it consumes you so much. Then the next stage is your silence, you don't want to talk to anyone but just sit in front of the TV and zone out. Don't worry! This is common, when your body gets blocked and also affects your mental health. I can get you out of your monkey toxic brain, as I have the formula on how to do it. I have been doing male brain chemicals for many years and the beautiful herbal tonics and teas available to 'calm the farm' are amazing.

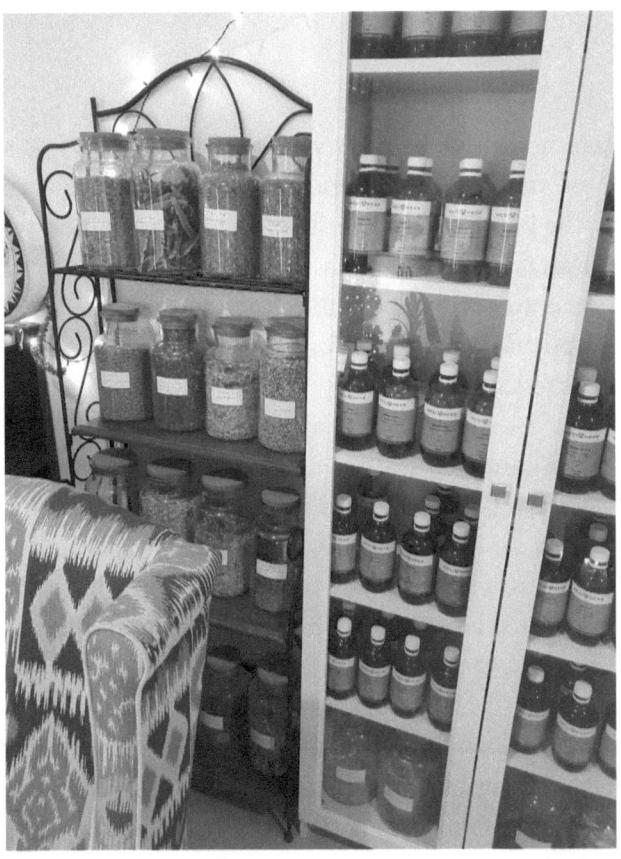

Endermologie® for men has a protocol that can help instantly release the toxins, coal dust and get the body moving. I like to promote flushing of the cerebrospinal fluid up the spine into the brain with the rollers using a roll in and roll out technique. My male clients can be so blocked, they instantly fall asleep in the hour treatment. This sleep can be so deep, as the body is so exhausted it just needs to switch completely off while detoxing. Each week seeing the difference from the man first coming in that is exhausted, fatigued, short tempered to a man that is now energised, happy, doing more activities with his family. I just get so excited when they say I'm getting along with my wife now and I feel less stressed! Whoopee! I do the happy dance.

Gout

Gout is common in men and is very painful to have. It is when the body has too much uric acid and this can cause it to crystallise in the joints. The joints will have inflammation and redness with severe pain. Gout attacks can come on suddenly usually at night and the common areas are the big toe, ankle, knee and fingers. To reduce uric acid; avoid purine-rich foods, sugar, alcohol, increase fibre, reduce weight and stress.

Once at band camp no really, once I had a client that his toe was nearly black from gout that it was ready to be chopped off. I put him on a foot detox and the tissue on the toe slowly split and this gunk just oozed out, it was so fascinating. We changed his diet, reduced alcohol and flushed his system with endermologie® and thermal wraps. He recovered and was able to keep the toe.

Avoiding excess alcohol can be difficult as it is often self-medicating. The client is feeling low and turns to alcohol to numb them as it's similar to a depressant. If we can use herbs to calm the system and feel good, then it is less of an issue to reduce alcohol. My 'happy juice' herbs are *Scutellaria lateriflora, Hypericum perforatum, Matricaria recutita, Passiflora incarnata* to name a few.

My gout herbs I love are *Centella asiatica, Apium graveolens, Ginkgo biloba, Calendula officinalis* to also name a few. I also love manuka honey for the wound and cherry juice on an empty stomach with folate, lots of folate. One time I even used a potato poultice that had great benefits. And water, water, water! These herbs need to be taken at different stages of gout, so please see your qualified practitioner.

Lactic Acid Build-up

Uric acid is not the same as lactic acid. Lactic acid build-up in the body can happen because there is not enough oxygen in the muscles and it creates a fermentation. It's not a bad thing, it's just usually from excessive exercise. We need this to break down our sugars in the body that are called glucose and glycogen that is needed for our ATP energy. Lactic acid is when our cells produce energy with intense exercise but without enough oxygen. Without oxygen, the cells will need to use a different energy source and our muscles and red blood cells dump it there. So really if you're creating too much lactic acid in your body by training excessively and your body is not riding of it, you don't have enough oxygen to keep up with the excessive exercise and lactic build-up, then the signs in your body are muscle pain, cramps and fatigue, it is giving you warning signals, give me more oxygen. You ignore it, then your poor liver that is your biggest rubbish bin in your body, has to go to work overtime. Who likes overtime, when you're not even getting paid for it? Exercise isn't the only cause, it can be alcohol, its heart and liver issues, low blood sugar and yes, lack of oxygen. More importantly, lactic acid is found in our beers, wines, pickled and fermented foods, all those yummy man-foods.

I often get men that are in constant muscle pain, or kidney, liver issues due to the lactic acid build-up. There are two types of lactic acid L-lactate and D-lactate, with L-lactate being the most common one. When there is too much L-lactate this causes problems to the liver and the kidneys, as they are unable to remove the excess acid, such as alcohol that increases phosphate and acid levels and also impacts the kidneys. (2018 Whelan Corey) Often we hear about alkaline/acid levels in the body and this is due to the imbalance in the acid and the pH level.

Working with some of the top sports people over the years, the lactic acid build-up under the rollers can feel like cement. The endermologie® protocol helps treat hamstrings and calves, due to wearing work-boots all day, sitting behind a desk, or lactic acid build-up from intense exercise. When I release the acid, it can feel like rice-bubbles popping and is instant relief for the client. I can feel the suppleness come back instantly into the tissue and muscles, reduce bloating in the gut and reduce aching joints and therefore less likely to get injured in sport.

Oxygen

Now let's talk about lack of oxygen in the blood. Low blood oxygen levels can cause shortness of breath, headaches, restlessness, dizziness, chest pain, confusion and high blood pressure. We breathe in through our lungs and the oxygen is collected by the red blood cells and delivered to parts of our body. You can use a pulse oximeter to check on oxygen levels and anything below 60mm Hg is considered unhealthy. (2020 Murrell Daniel) There are many causes but the major cause out here is the coal dust. We need to keep the lungs healthy and free of debris build-up. So, we need to breathe fresh air, open up those windows, but obviously not out west here as it's too hot and dusty, so instead fill your house with oxygen rich plants and eat iron-rich foods to promote more oxygen to be transported from the lungs in our blood. Use an air purifier filter machine in your bedroom when you sleep. I really love the Hepa filters. Have an endermologie® treatment weekly to promote oxygen in your blood by 400% blood circulation and flush the lungs and lymphatic system out.

Testosterone

Hormones are a topic I often treat with men. I'm constantly asked how can I increase my testosterone? Or 'I'm tired all the time', muscle wasting, low sex drive and feeling depleted. The secret to testosterone building is easy. Take the toxins out of the body that are blocking the body from producing testosterone. Exercise and lift weights, eat protein, fat and carbs, get some sun or take Vitamin D and minimise stress and your cortisol levels. Low testosterone can cause fatigue, mood changes and it can make it difficult to get and maintain erections because testosterone stimulates the penile tissues. Often, it snow-balls later to increased body fat around the gut and loss of muscle fat and worse, decreased bone mass. This is similar to women going through menopause, men can go through male menopause early, if they are toxic, it's as traumatic to the body and mind.

Endermologie® is the missing link treatment for men to detox their body, stop cravings for comfort foods, allowing the body to naturally build testosterone as the digestive system improves, reduce gut overload and give definition to the muscles. As a herbalist the natural plant food enhancing testosterone tonics, teas and supplements are also a huge success.

> 'Take care of your body. It's the only place you have to live'
> **-Jim Rohn**

CHAPTER 6

Thyroid

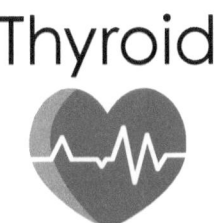

'Am I the only one that can go to the gym 5 days a week and actually gain weight'

-hypothyroidmom.com

Has your thyroid been giving you issues? Are you constantly fighting the horrible side effects of either your medication or the hideous symptoms of thyroid issues?

Endermologie® is to the rescue, for a treatment that increases your blood circulation in your body by 400%, to increase your lymph system to finally kick into gear and pump your waste and garbage out. The thyroid protocol is the body treatment followed by a face treatment to give a complete complex thyroid protocol to help flush your thyroid.

The thyroid protocol flushes up through the lungs into the thyroid promoting healthy blood flow. The thyroid loves blood flow and the lymphatic flush as it helps promote the reduction of inflammation of the thyroid. I then use a separate small head that rolls up gently and over the thyroid to also flush the left/right lymph glands as well. The lymphatic drainage of the thyroid drains into the superior deep cervical nodes, so these nodes get a complete endermologie® flush.

While the body treatment helps release all the lymph and increase blood circulation, the face detox protocol specialises in the drainage of the thyroid and also includes a neck flush. The results can be amazing! Excess fluid in the neck removed instantly and draining of the thyroid area leaving a more prominent jawline. The entire face reduces in puffiness and gets a natural face-lift, as a bonus.

The thyroid is located just below the Adam's-apple and just above the clavicle bone and is made up of two lobes. The thyroid is part of our endocrine system that is made up of nine glands – Hypothalamus, Pineal Gland, Pituitary Gland, Parathyroid, Thymus, Adrenal, Pancreas, Ovaries, Testes and the Thyroid. These glands release hormones that regulate and keep our body in check. Our thyroid is crucial to our body, as it regulates our heart rate, body weight, muscle strength, breathing, nervous system, energy and basically everything.

The thyroid releases two hormones called Triiodothyronine (T3) and Thyroxine (T4) and these hormones regulate the metabolism of our body. When too much of these hormones are released, the cells in our body are working overtime causing Hyperthyroidism. If our body becomes lazy and doesn't release enough of these hormones into the body, we slow down, it is called Hypothyroidism.

Hypothyroidism

Hypothyroidism is the metabolic rate and the body slowing down on you. The symptoms are tiredness, feeling cold, weight gain, depression and lack of concentration. Sometimes we don't even know we have it, as it can be more common in older women that think it's just part of ageing with dry skin, weight gain and even constipation. We become fatigued and can lose our mental clarity and become quite foggy and this makes it hard to tell it apart from other health issues, such as menopause.

A slow metabolism and slow thyroid is going to feel like you're dragging your feet. Sometimes your thyroid can enlarge and produce a goitre, that is like an enlarged lump. There are certain foods you need to avoid and supplements you need to take for this. Over the years of treating so many clients I have found even if they eat and take their supplements, the endermologie® is needed to kick-back their body into gear. I usually need a programme of twelve treatments and a Herbal/Naturopath consultation. Once the thyroid is at a healthy level depending on age, a maintenance of fortnightly to a month is needed.

Hyperthyroidism

Hyperthyroidism is totally different; it's all about the body going too fast. The symptoms are weight-loss, can't stand the heat, anxiety, irritated eyes that are itchy or gritty and very anxious. Even sensitivity to noises, jumpy feeling that can get you turned on all the time. Also, you are so wired up, you can have sleep issues, then impatience and irritability. All these symptoms can also cross over between the two hyper and hypo thyroidism, just to confuse you.

Thyroid Hormones

So, we know the thyroid gland produces T3 and T4 hormones and releases into the bloodstream. The thyroid needs iodine from foods to make these two hormones. The thyroid cells also need one more amino acid to mix with the iodine called tyrosine to make the T3 and T4. Then T3 T4 off they go through our bloodstream where they are in charge of our metabolism and to keep us active. Keep with me on this as this is the most important part.

Metabolism also converts oxygen and calories to energy! So basically, your fat is being used or 'burned' to rev your body up, if your thyroid is working properly. Often, I supplement with the treatments and I also mix a thyroid tonic up to take while having the endermologie® treatments, just to have the complete protocol for excellent results.

Blood Tests

When I order your bloods for your thyroid, I will test for T3, T4, TSH and antibodies. You understand why the T3 and T4 need to be tested, but let me explain the other two important tests needed. T4 produces about 80% of the hormone even though T3 produces 20%, it's nearly four times in strength and very strong. Now these hormones love the heat and this is why you can feel cold with hypothyroidism and hot with hyperthyroidism.

Another gland in the endocrine system is the pituitary gland that produces thyroid stimulating hormone (TSH) that controls T4 and T3 so testing TSH is important too.

The final test for the thyroid is the antibodies, to test if there is an autoimmune thyroid disease. (TPO antibodies) This could be Graves Disease or Hashimotos.

Great news! These readings in your blood work can all be balanced with tonics, supplements, change of diet and endermologie®.

Oxalates

Oxalates can also be the root cause of thyroid issues, so it's important for me to bring up the cause of oxalates and how they affect the thyroid. There are three components, oxalates, calcium and iron. Oxalates and lack of calcium can cause inflammation in your tissues; with a mixture of iron you get oxidative damage, iron levels decrease and cause fatigue. These oxalates can get in your thyroid and give you huge issues and can possibly be part of the cause of your thyroid issues.

Our body can usually break down the oxalates in the gut with oxalate genes, but if these genes have been compromised the oxalates can't get broken down and passed through the urine or stools. Stress…welcome to everyone's world, your gut lining and good bacteria breaks down and you are unable to break down the oxalates. When you dump excess oxalates the issues can be; hives, developmental disorders in children, kidney stones, leaky gut, chelating toxic metals, depression, vulvodynia, burning bowel movements, cystitis, inflamed joints, rheumatoid arthritis, lupus, fibromyalgia and most important thyroid issues. (2019 Mercola, Joseph)

When you have high oxalate foods, you can also have a DNA issue when your oxalate genes are not working properly and can create an excess of the oxalate crystals. These crystals are like razor sharp that can get in your joints, tissues, lungs, kidneys and your thyroid and cause major problems. I have had many clients come in with lower back pain. Often this is high oxalates in the kidneys and when treated the pain will go.

I have many clients coming in with thyroid issues and have put so much weight on and have become puffy like a bull-frog and their toe nails can be of grey appearance, that is also a significant sign.

Their mind-set is so anxious and worried all the time and they are really struggling with life, being so intense all the time and just not

Endermologie®

feeling good about themselves and their weight-issues. I immediately put them on my programme of endermologie® to flush their thyroid of possible oxalates and kick their body back into gear. I then give an amazing herbal tonic I designed up, that is natural plant food to kick the thyroid hormones T3, T4, TSH back into gear. Also, we swap their foods, take supplements and help the thyroid back to a healthy normal state.

'To keep the body in good health is a duty...otherwise we shall not be able to keep the mind strong and clear'
-Buddha

CHAPTER 7

Fertility

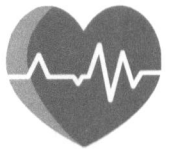

'You might have to fight a battle more than once to win it'

-Margaret Thatcher

Have you been trying to get pregnant? It's so frustrating with the waiting game and the disappointments. Or even worse, have you been getting pregnant and having miscarriages? The pain of trying to recover is hideous.

I have so many clients coming to see me about fertility. It is one of my most popular endermologie® treatments I do. I really get excited and rewarded when I first start treating infertility and then it follows through to their pregnancy and I wait patiently to see the new bub.

Fertility Treatment

The endermologie® treatment I do for fertility, uses a technique that flushes. It promotes lots of blood flow to the ovaries to flush them out and promote the healthy blood flow to heal the tissue. The rollers mobilize the tissues for an awakening. You can feel the organs being drained of toxins that prevent the body from doing their natural process for fertility. Draining the liver also, is important to rid the body of all the toxic oestrogens that can cause serious health issues.

The rollers roll in and roll out causing a mechanical stimulation of the cells to actually wake them up and promote new healthy cellular growth. Some ladies may fall pregnant after the first treatment or some may need the four months in that time for the dormant cellular activity to be replaced with new healthy cells.

Often, when I run over their stomach, I can feel the blockages. They are actually lumpy and you can feel the rollers breaking them up. The satisfaction you can feel when the rollers run freely through the gut, allowing fresh healthy blood to go to work and heal the organs, especially the ovaries.

I had one lady that had been trying for over a year to get pregnant, booked in for foot endo and wrap with me and disappeared. I found out later, only after one treatment that she had fallen pregnant straight away. Of course, everyone is different and their body is at different stages. Now that same client is back for her second baby. This time I am asking her to wait until her baby body is back to its original toned tight healthy state and free of all toxins, so her eggs are also healthy and her pregnancy will be complication free. I do get a kick out of seeing all the baby pics though. Or even better, I see the little ones at Coles when I go shopping.

Infertility and MTHFR

Let's talk about synthetic Folic Acid that is being put in our foods and a lot of us have no idea it's being done. The Government has been supplementing our foods in Australia with synthetic Folic Acid to help with birth defects. The problem is there is no regulation to how much we consume and it can affect our major gene in the body. This major gene affects all our genes in our body causing issues with fertility. The gene is called Methylenetetrahydrofolate (MTHFR). MTHFR is an enzyme in our body that converts folic acid into a usable form but if this gene is compromised, it can lead to backing up of an amino acid homocysteine that is toxic to the body.

Folic acid is a man-made supplement, it's a synthetic form of folate that is being added to all fortified foods such as; white flour goods, cakes, biscuits, cereals and even our supplements and protein powders. Folate is completely different; it is Vitamin B9 and is found naturally in our foods. Often people can have genes that due to high synthetic Folic Acid intake prevents the natural Folate from being absorbed.

I just love DNA and froth over genes. Get me talking about them and I won't stop. It's like going into another world, so I will try to keep it as simplified as possible. There is a pathway in our DNA that the folate needs to go through in the body and it has many steps to help it get converted into the active form of folate 5-MTHFR. Now the MTHFR gene is right at the end of the pathway, so if any of the other genes are turned off or not working correctly this can affect your fertility issues. If these genes are not working correctly your body can't absorb foods, vitamins and nutrients needed to help you get pregnant. A DNA complete analysis also allows you to see your MTHFR pathway and any issues associated with your infertility issues along the way.

Our average daily intake of Folic Acid should be 200-400 mcg but if we have excess fortified white flour foods; we can increase it to

800-1000 mcg, well over our required intake. This goes on for years building up in our system, our DNA will change and affect our major gene the MTHFR.

Folate is what we get from our vegetables and is part of the B-Vitamins and it helps make red and white blood cells in the bone marrow and produces our DNA. It's the good stuff. The problem is we don't absorb enough folate, our unhealthy lifestyles of packaged fortified foods and lack of fresh organic vegetables reduces our MTHFR gene that is vital in fertility. It is important to do a DNA analysis of your genes to find out if your fertility pathway is working correctly. To do this, I prefer the www.ancestory.com to test genes as they have a broad range of genes included. I do two forms of DNA test: a short test for the MTHFR gene or a complete test that can take up to two weeks.

Toxicity

A lot of my clients feel as if they are celiac because they can't cope with the gluten and come to me with stomach issues. Sometimes they eat certain foods and it reacts, then other times they eat the same foods and it's all good. The gut issues can be from excess synthetic Folic Acid, pesticides on foods, food colourings, packaged foods with additives to name a few. Then we top it off with eating wheat products and foods being sprayed with glyphosate that can kill our gut bacteria that gives us the stomach and bowel issues. Then we drink water with fluoride, put deodorants that contain aluminium, parabens, store our food in plastics, our poor body is blocked up with toxins.

By the time my clients come to me, their poor DNA needs the groundwork put in to start healing all the damage done to their fertility pathway, heavy metal toxicity overload and possibly the major cause of their infertility. This is from everyday living and on top of it, in our town we have our coal dust issues. My clients realise to live here in Moranbah, they need to detox at least once a month, if they have no health issues or weekly to fortnightly if they do, to keep their health at an optimal level.

It doesn't have to be in the mines either, as an example of environmental toxicity currently in the USA, thousands of people are coming forward with litigation. This extract is from the New York Times. 'An agreement to pay more than $10 billion to settle thousands of claims that the popular weed killer Roundup causes cancer is unravelling.' (2020 Patricia Cohen) Our everyday convenient household products and what is being used to spray our foods with can be causing cancer is a huge worry.

Endermologie® is needed with the environmental toxicity we take in daily to flush it out. Our cells feel a huge sigh of relief when the toxicity is detoxed out safely. Detoxing safely is important; as one client came to see me after they did their own detox from reading on the Internet, a home gall bladder cleanse; this caused large stones to block and ended up having to take the gall bladder out. It is so important to encapsulate toxins so when you detox them out, they don't go into the blood stream and make you very sick or reduce the stones down to gravel before you pass them.

I have had many successful ladies this year conceive. It's been a hard journey for some when they first arrive to see me, as they come after one or more miscarriages and healing mentally and emotionally is a huge challenge. Building that confidence back up and changing their foods and their lifestyle so they are happy again is also so satisfying.

On the opposite scale, I actually have to warn all my female clients to be aware as you could possibly become fertile even if you haven't for years, with endermologie®. One client had never been pregnant in her life and was 48 years old and fell pregnant within four endermologie® sessions that was a shock to her. Another, in her late thirties also never been able to conceive had totally given up trying, also fell pregnant. The missing link to infertility is possibly endermologie® to plump and renew your cells but also to balance out your DNA to conceive and give birth, using tonics, herbal teas, supplements and nutrition.

'A baby is something you carry inside you for nine months, in your arms for three years, and in your heart until the day you die.'

-Mary Mason.

SUMMARY

Part One

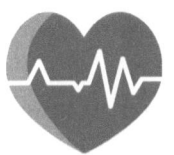

Endermologie® is one of the most important treatments you can do to help heal your health and to live a happy fulfilled life. It is a valuable component to empower you to overcome your weight and obesity issues that have been causing you so much heartache. In our crazy times with a pandemic, we are all realising how important our health is, it can save our lives, by being healthy. The increase in health issues and even more with our children are increasing so much. The losing battle of crazy diets can stop now and endermologie® can get you back on track to a slim, energised body that you deserve. I can teach you how easy it is to lose a kilo a week with your dedication and drive to achieve your goals or to keep your body, mind and emotions balanced by detoxing once a month.

The number of mental health issues is increasing every year. The endermologie® protocol helps to pull you out of your funk and into a happy healthy life. How good would it be for you to leap out of bed with energy in the morning?

Don't let menopause rule your life with your fluctuating moods and basically being mean to the people around you. Take control of your hormones and do not allow them to rule your life. Learn to empower yourself, by flushing out your ovaries and renewing your energy and vitality in your body.

To all the Mums and Dads out there, your children's health is so important to set a great foundation up for your child now, so they don't have health issues later on in their adult life. Or to help improve their behaviour, concentration and focus at school or more important to have a happy childhood. Children play up when their body is blocked with toxins and they have a tendency to copy their parent's health habits.

Men are now looking for ways to improve their health, to improve the way they feel. Men's health is important, so they can go to work and not feel fatigued at the end of the day, to reduce fogginess, to have mental clarity and to finally have control of fluctuating moods of anger, frustration and being overwhelmed. Also, to help with their sex drive as they are losing their testosterone due to heavy metal toxicity, especially out here in the coal mines due to the coal dust. The endermologie® protocol for a man is amazing. The results each week show how energised, but calm they can become and able to tackle situations in their life with a big bonus, with their gut reducing in size.

Then, there is the cost on your health not to heal your thyroid with the constant debilitating symptoms that keep coming back. Or the frustrations of not being able to conceive. Endermologie® protocols used in conjunction with my other machines, tonics, supplements, herbal teas, DNA, exercise and sound therapy meditation, can help you to overcome these conditions.

Endermologie® can perhaps give you hope to believe in yourself, believe you can win so many health struggles because if you have absolute certainty you can beat your health issues, you will! We also work on your state of mind to improve in your belief system and create challenges in your life that are so rewarding. I use a combination of the Hoffman Process, Psychosynthesis psychology and counselling methods I am qualified in to help improve your mindset. Oh and Tony Robbins workshops I am such a huge fan and have put many of my clients onto.

If your spouse is back at home, eating ice-cream and junk food it's hard on you to not also join in, but your strong state of mind can beat the urges of unhealthy eating and usually the whole family will get on board when they see how well you are doing. It is so exciting when the family joins in as a unit you can make it a game with the children, they can have fun learning to eat new foods and their complimentary crystal I give after each treatment also encourages them.

It's a process I take you through but it's a simple process that you can follow, it's not complicated but the weight-loss each week takes the pressure of your body to heal your thyroid and increase your fertility but most of all endermologie® gives you the secret to looking good but feel amazing!

I need your time and your attention to mould you into a healthy lifestyle that is easy to follow. It's not just about you losing weight, it's about you changing your life. This is why I'm doing this because I devote my life to changing your life, it is my passion that gets results. This is the key to endermologie®, it's what I do! It's about taking the time to book in and take your energy and your health to the next level. To get out of being stuck in your unhealthy lifestyle. It's your launchpad to feeling happy, energized and the freedom to be successful in all aspects of your life. How often have you noticed, when you feel healthy everything goes right in your life? You think positively, you make positive goals to achieve and suddenly you are around positive people.

The Ultimate 5-day Retreat

As I live remotely, I have had to design a 5-day package up for clients that move away or for clients with health issues that need strong treatments. This is for clients that need to seriously change their health or need a huge push into getting a healthy mind and body back. As an example, I had a lady come up from Melbourne before Coronavirus, for the five-day package for Chronic Fatigue. This poor dear would get up in the morning, shower and have to lie down on the couch after being totally fatigued just from doing those few morning tasks. By the fifth day, I had her swimming, bike-riding and walking every day. Her whole life changed completely and she was able to go home and do activities with her children and husband that was not possible for years. Living remotely is a huge part of the success in this package as there are no distractions while you are here, you are totally focused. You are required to complete the four-hour treatments daily involving four machines and the sound bowls. Then your day will consist of food swaps, herbal tonics, teas with activities of meditation, yoga, swimming and PT sessions depending on the client's health to complete their challenge.

My Ultimate Experience Package is your path to your freedom to a healthy body and a healthy mind. Whether it's chronic fatigue, thyroid issues, infertility, anxiety, depression or gaining control of your weight, it's your next step to freedom to a healthy body at last. I will walk you through step-by-step in making those changes that are baby steps and so easy to achieve. This package involves you stepping up each day to make your changes in your health. Never have to diet again, never have to go through that pain of feeling you're missing out on food. Food is glorious, it's a social part of our lives that we embrace with our families. It's part of sitting down with the family each night and talking about your day at the table without being glued to your mobile phone. Let me take you on your endermologie® path to the secret, to look good, feel good and achieve the 'Wow' factor.

'Opportunities don't happen. You create them'
-Chris Grosser

PART TWO

The Therapist

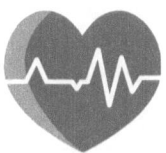

'Always deliver more than expected'

-**Larry Page**

CHAPTER 8
Endermologie® Machines

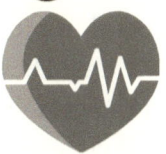

This second half of the book, I am going to share with you my experiences as a therapist with the endermologie® machine, so you will have the confidence to be a machine guru also. Even though the endermologie® machine basically runs itself, I am going to empower you as a therapist so you will be in awe as to what you can do to help your clients health with this amazing machine and take it to the next level. First of all, you need to name it. Mine is 'Charlie' and all the clients call it Charlie and relate to it as their saviour and they have a personal experience with him of pure bliss. They know Charlie is going to finally make them feel happy and look good, by improving all their health issues.

The Cellu M6® Alliance is the latest generation machine and I have the medical grade one that looks very space-age and is able to get instant results. This machine provides a natural cell stimulation and rejuvenation process that clinics all around the world have been using. In this book, I have taken it to the next level with all my medical research and my personal experience over the years that will encourage more therapists to use this machine. I am one of the oldest operators in the world, with over 20 years in the business, to help heal the body of disease. I am going to teach you how you can also jump on board and bring this machine into your business to be so successful and even continue on throughout pandemics and GFC as I did, earning a living in helping your clients to heal, detox and change their way of life.

The French

The machine was first designed in 1983 by Louis Paul Guitay, a French engineer. Mr Guitay was involved in a terrible car accident with burn injuries and muscle damage. He found he had to have hours of massage to help his healing process and so he designed the first endermologie® machine to heal burns and scar victims. He started a family business called LPG® and so began the story of endermologie® treatments that is world-wide now.

The Machines
The Cellu M6® Keymodule [2]i

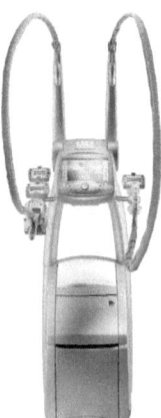

Cellu M6®Keymodule (2)I
©LPG systems 2020

Endermologie® Machines

The first machine I got was the Cellu M6® Keymodule [2]i and it lasted me for over 15 years. Then a new technology machine range came in and I must admit I didn't want to change over, as my results were amazing and nothing could be better than my old Charlie. I really dug my heels in and was so angry I had to change to a new machine. How could they do this to me! Yet how silly of me.

The Cellu M6® Integral[2]

But I was so wrong! I finally gave in and purchased the Cellu M6® Integral[2]. This machine is ideal for the therapist that is serious about endermologie® and is willing to take the time to train. This machine was so much stronger and efficient, I couldn't believe it. The results I was getting instead of needing 14 treatments, were in 4 treatments! It was so smooth to use I could feel the skin, tissue, organs even better through the rollers than my old machine. I was a little frustrated at the beginning as we now have to hold the head with two hands wrapped around the head but soon realised this gave my wrists more support and less likely to ache after 10 hours a day doing treatments.

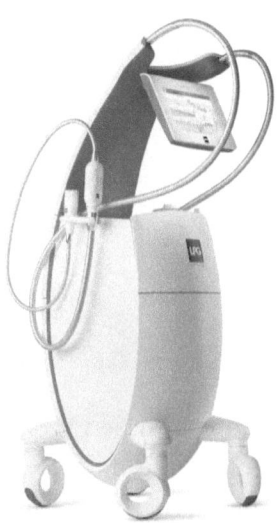

Cellu M6® Integral
©LPG systems 2020

The Cellu M6® Alliance

Now, because I had left it so long to purchase the Cellu M6® Integral[2] machine, another new machine came out called the Cellu M6® Alliance. This machine did all three movements in one go and you could go so high with absolutely no pain. I love both machines but keeping up with the newest technology is a must, but I still have both, I just couldn't let go of my last one.

On one side of the Cellu M6® Alliance machine is the body treatment, using the TH80 head that I use on most clients. It is interchangeable with the small head, the Alliance 50. I use this for smaller parts of the body, injuries, burns, scars and children's treatments.

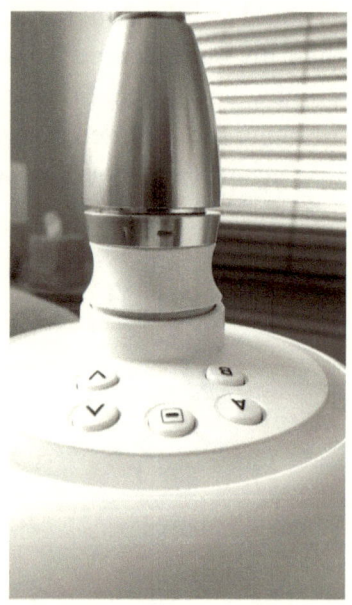

The other side of the machine has the Ergolift head that is used for the face, neck, décolleté and breast-lift. I use the Ergolift in my Face Detox protocol. Also, on this side of the machine is the interchangeable TR30 head that I use to treat temporomandibular joint issues, (TMJ) burns, scars, feet issues such as plantar fasciitis, Achilles tendon injury and cramping.

Endermologie® Machines

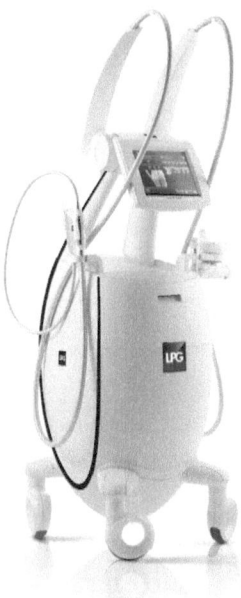

Cellu M6® Alliance
©LPG systems 2020

The Cellu M6® Alliance is for you, if you have no experience as it tells you what moves to do and when. With the purchase of each machine, you are required to complete a training course. It is a very simple machine to use. The face treatment gives you a face-lift, increases collagen and elastin, plumps your lips without injectables but most of all which I get so excited about, it detoxes! Over the years I have designed for myself detox protocols for different health issues and now I want to share with Naturopaths, Herbalists and health practitioners to incorporate with their consultations to flush out embedded toxins that block our DNA pathways. A client has one Naturopath consultation and then follow-up consultations if needed. Endermologie® is an ongoing weekly treatment to keep the body healing and kick-start it into optimal health. Often the client won't make changes to their health or lifestyles, as it is all too hard. As a therapist I have found giving supplements, herbal tonics, teas or nutritional plans are just not enough to get the client immediate results to feel good. Also, there are some clients that just don't follow through. Endermologie® steps in and gives the clients a big kick start and motivates them to change their habits.

The detox protocol I have designed up is the new Face Detox procedure, as out here in the mines the coal dust particles can cause many nasal, ear and eye issues. If you are interested, continue reading as I have a chapter further on with a step-by-step guide on how to do the new Face Detox procedure.

The Cellu M6® Alliance machine has a head that uses rollers to pick up the tissue and then roll in and roll out to drain, tone and detox. The name of the procedure is called endermologie.® The blood circulation is increased by 400% and this causes the lymph system to start moving, that is the main cause of a lot of health issues. As a therapist we are always trying to detox the liver, gall bladder, kidneys and flush the lymph system with supplements and exercise, but it can take time and clients now want instant results. They are always looking for something that is quick. Endermologie® can deliver and the great thing is you get to see your client more often and check to see they are following through with their tonics, supplements, lifestyle changes and also see if something needs to be tweaked. Sometimes as a therapist, clients may not tell you a supplement or food plan is not suitable and they just won't come back. This way, having regular endermologie® sessions everything can be discussed and re-evaluated during each treatment.

Here are some tips you may be interested in.

Tip one; training on how to use the machine. I have used it over the years with many therapists. Close your eyes when you are treating a client; it is an amazing experience. You can clearly feel the client's tissue and organs as you move through the body, you can feel the blockages and the satisfaction of feeling the blockages move. It is a great way to connect to their body.

Endermologie® Machines

Tip two; is to do an hour treatment on the client breaking it up into two 30 minute continuous treatments. Every treatment I start with the back protocol going up the spine into the neck, this instantly relaxes the client and makes your job easier at releasing the blockages. Men especially go into a deep sleep. By the second round on the back, trying to turn them over is a challenge as I need to look out for arms or legs that can jerk when woken up, while women tend to go into a floating experience and can't talk.

Tip three; when the client is in this state, don't talk. This is the best experience your client can ever have. It's the complete nervous system letting go and finally relaxing that monkey brain that never shuts up. It's similar to the feeling when you have just completed a yoga session and you are in a dream state.

Tip four; keep yourself fit. I have seen over the years therapists having to give up due to back ache or wrist pain. I have never experienced any of this and this is because my morning ritual in the gym is lifting weights for wrist strength and sit-ups daily for strength in the back. Heck, I'm 57 years of age and I have a little six-pack from doing endermologie®. Also, you need to walk the talk and be healthy. How can you recommend to your clients to live a healthy lifestyle if you are not doing it? I have my naughty times occasionally and have something sweet or a gluten free pizza but then I get back on track and follow through by eating healthy, exercising and doing treatments on myself. Yes, you can do endermologie® on yourself and I totally recommend it, I have been doing it for years every week and I have really slowed my ageing process down because of it, as I'm not storing toxins in my body and my skin loves it.

Tip five; keep your treatment table high with your knees bent and rock back and forth sideways so you don't lock your hips in. I went and did a Kahuna massage course to learn to move when I am treating as my hips would ache at the end of the day, this helped immensely.

Maintenance Filters

The maintenance on this machine is easy. The endermologie® machine have filters in the back that are easy to access with a draw that opens up. One side is for the face and one side is for the body. It is important to constantly vacuum these out, as they collect all the skin and fluff up of the client's suit.

Tip six; never use towels on your treatment table with the client lying directly on them as they get fluff on them and block the machine. I always use a fresh crisp sheet for each client, even the paper roles can get particles up in them.

The machine also exfoliates the skin, so the particles of skin get sucked up through the machine and collect in the filters. Years ago, I wasn't told this and I soon found out that if I would blow into the treatment head to clear it, the skin particles would go up into my face. Urrg!

Tip seven; do not blow onto the head of the machine or where the filters go in, as this is all your clients skin build-up, it is not fluff and not hygienic to go up into your face!

The filters are replaced when a light comes on of a spanner on the machine, to let you know it's time to change them, which is every 250 hours. Every time I change my filter I celebrate and do a happy dance as I have achieved an income and helped so many clients, change their health. Then every two years, or 1000 hours, you get an endermologie® technician in to service it. That is it! easy-peasy!

Plastic Flaps

The head of the body machine has plastic flaps that need to be changed and cleaned. (Link to show you how… https://www.youtube.com/

watch?v=X3z66ffMJgs&list=PLrBOG_nruLe2Zt1rpgARVIAl6gjiSB3Ya&index=6)

With the different heads on the machine, you can also incorporate different treatments for more variety of clientele. Over the years I have treated burns, scars, fibrosis or thickening of skin due to injury, accidents or plastic surgery. I often use the smaller head for pre and post operative procedures. Working closely with the client's surgeon, we are able to prepare the tissue before the operation to help with less bruising and infection. After the operation, drainage with butterfly heads to softly flush the site with healthy blood flow and promote tissue to heal three times quicker. I am very busy with plastic surgery clients that are pre and post operative.

I am sad to say we have mine accidents out here in Moranbah and over the years I quietly track down the wives who have had family loss and give them free endermologie® to help them sleep and cope with their trauma.

Tip eight; put carpet down if you have a tiled floor. You will drop these heads and they will crack and they're costly to replace. I learnt this the hard way, yes I have dropped them, wooden floors and tiles are a nightmare.

The face machine also has flaps you use. These need to be sterilised after each use. The client can purchase their own face-kits (flaps) and bring them for each treatment but I stopped this due to health issues and COVID. I supply the flaps and I sterilise them each time after the treatment and again before the treatment. I also wipe them with disinfectant wipes during the treatment, in case particles get caught in the flaps. It is the same as the body stockings I supply them as I know I have washed and sterilised them correctly. I used to have clients leave them in their car and forget to wash them.

Transporting

Tip nine; it is important to put this machine on a trolly with wheels if transporting. Do not allow the removalists to wheel it on and leave it free standing on the truck. The legs cannot deal with the truck going over bumps and can snap. It must be supported and strapped down on a trolly with the wheels off the ground. This information will save you a lot of headaches over the years, if you have to move your clinic. Take off the handle by turning it slightly, then it lifts off. Wrap the machine in blankets. Then tie it down onto the trolley. I wish I had saved my box, what it came in.

Tip ten; save your box!

In each country, there is a distributor you have to go through to purchase one, you cannot purchase directly from France. Training is included and is basic for you to get started. The new Cellu M6 Alliance® is simple as you can follow everything on the screen. Eventually as your confidence grows, you will accommodate your client treating them for what they need, not so much for what the screen on your machine says. It is learning to understand all the organs in the body and the lymph system. If you want to learn to treat the body for health issues like me, you will need to have a background as a practitioner. If you want to treat beauty, then a beauty or massage training is ideal. The treatments I designed are incorporated with years of University study and research as a Herbalist, Naturopath and Nutritionist.

My 'Charlie' is amazing and over the years I have treated so many clients with different issues. Using these mechanical rollers to get that lymph system moving and breaking up blockages in the body is an amazing treatment to include within your clinic. My feedback from clients is; it makes them feel energised, healthier, slimmer, toned and motivated to eat better and start exercising.

CHAPTER 9

Psychology in Business

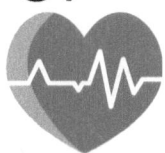

I have been my own boss for over 30 years. Being able to choose when I can work, or how much I need to work or more important when to stop work, has all been a learning curve for me. Being your own boss is amazing but you can become a workaholic and it's all about balance, especially learning how to say no to your clients and taking time off. It is about you yourself living a healthy lifestyle and following what you teach. Often business owners get burnt-out. We want to build our business to a success as this reflects on us personally. This can turn us into perfectionists or have OCD tendencies due to all the cleaning and sterilising.

Tip eleven; go do a course at least twice a year on self-development. I have Christian values but I am constantly working with people that have all sorts of issues and you need to learn to not take it on. I have completed heaps of Tony Robbins courses where I fire-walk every four years or chop wood in half to keep myself in a peak state. As well I have done the Mathew Hussey retreat, Hoffman Process, walked the PNG Kokoda trek, skydived even though I'm so terrified of heights, all to challenge myself. I have trained with two women Aboriginal Elders in women's issues, done an original Vision Quest with a Cherokee lady and learnt the ways of a Maori elder, all areas to help me open up to a cultural understanding and how we are all unique in our own special way.

My business has been through the GFC, when everyone was closing down in the world. It went through when the mine industry dropped through the bottom and everyone lost their jobs and now a world pandemic with the COVID, that is seeing many businesses close their doors. The secret to endermologie® is people need to feel good no matter what is happening in their lives and will search for treatments to achieve this. Wearing the enderowear™ also separates the therapist from touching the client in times of health restrictions and this is a bonus during COVID.

It is all about being flexible and understanding that your clients could be going through gunk that has been stuck causing fat cells and toxins to accumulate in the body, some for many years and now they are noticing. Moving this gunk can be emotional as your client has an attachment to it physically, spiritually or mentally and it's stuck in their cells.

Tip Twelve; turn up to work a 100% ready with a smile and energy that vibrates onto your client. Not giving the client sympathy if they are down, but giving them the truth to what they are doing to put themselves in that state. This is your most valuable tip of all. It doesn't matter if you have a new fancy clinic or spent thousands on a refit. It is all about hygiene, a clean clinic and the client has to connect with you and feel comfortable. Don't make your room too sterile but if a client can go to sleep in your treatment room it means your clinic is relaxing.

Endermologie® can change lives, it helps promote people to clear the fog out of their heads. I often get clients that come to me because their

GP has said, there is nothing wrong with them but the client knows and feels they are not at their optimal healthy state. When the client comes to you, they are often feeling low and you need to take over and assure them they are in the right place. Endermologie® kick starts people onto a new healthy path, not only physically but emotionally and mentally with the help of your positive energy.

When clients come to you blocked physically, mentally and emotionally, you will need to start out slow. We need to release enough toxins to unblock and start to feel amazing between 1-3 days later after the treatment. Sometimes you need to pull back and detox slowly. I don't treat clients on heavy drugs, like ice and recommend you do not do this at all, that is a completely different area, that professional detox centres are going to help with their problem. Detoxing heavy drugs with endermologie® and machines can make the client very sick.

When a client comes in my door, I am bright and breezy every single time. I leave behind my own personal garbage and I put my work hat on and get to business.

You need to also learn to smell the release of the different toxins coming out of your client's body. An example is mold, it has its own distinct smell. Clients can have mold issues and spores in their body from living in houses that have flooded, as mold can be hidden all throughout the walls in the house. Learning to smell is important as it helps you also to treat correctly. Another example is eating lots of sugar and unbalancing their micro-bacteria in the body causing yeast and candida overgrowth is also a distinct older smell. These are areas you need to investigate by asking the right questions and being able to smell the toxicity coming out of the body and identifying with it, to find the correct endermologie® protocol to follow for that health issue. This is where I start with a Herbalist consultation combined with the treatments to get a holistic approach to healing their health.

Morning Prep

As I stated, I start my day by exercising every morning making sure I get in my peak state. You can't turn up at the door to welcome your client if you are tired, they can see straight through you. I exercise and drink two bottles of lemon water to flush my liver before I start the day. I then meditate or listen to my sound bowls, this process is so important. I have been meditating for over 40 years. It takes only a few minutes each morning to go within and centre myself. It is vital that you have strong mental and emotional clarity to cope with your client's issues that may arise. I learnt the hard way when I first started out. I completely crashed and ended up in bed with fatigue. It was because I took on all my client's 'garbage' they were dumping and it burnt me out. Now I can listen and never feel drained at the end of the day.

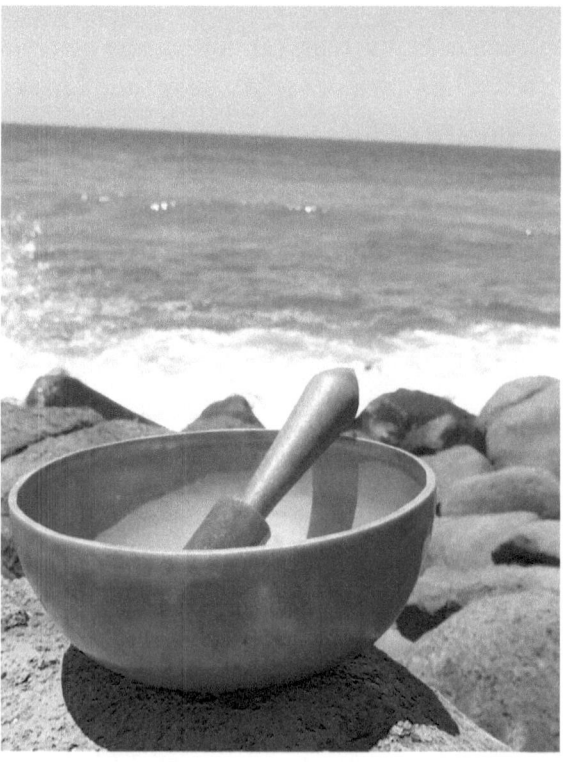

I also use Sound Therapy to help put me into a meditative state without even trying. I just want you to succeed as I have. Setting the groundwork up for your business is what is going to make you successful. As your emotional and spiritual energy increases, you will find you will get clients that are also on your level. I now get clients that are healers and treat other people. One client I had was a friend of the Dalai Lama and what an experience to treat her. Listen to your body, the sensations and feelings you get will give you messages to how your client needs to be treated.

Uniform

After you have prepped yourself with exercise and meditation, the next step is to dress yourself as a professional. I wear pants as you need to be squatting all the time and I wear a white shirt. I believe a white shirt is important as its clean and a crisp colour that signifies health. Also, if you wear colours some clients may not relate to your choice of colour perhaps when they are feeling sick or in a low mood. You need to wear tops that are stretchy tight so the sleeves don't get in your way and drape over the client when you lean over. Put your hair up and full make-up done. Nails done and clean tidy footwear. I use Orthaheel shoes as you are on your feet daily. The reason why I say put your hair up is not only because you are leaning forward over the client and your hair will get in the way but because at the end of the day; let your hair down, take your uniform off, shower with sandalwood soap to wash of all the energy of your day away and this lets your subconscious mind know you are now finished work. I also often sage my room to clear the energy of the room and open the windows to allow fresh air to flow.

Room Set-Up

Setting up your room is also important. You don't want a sterile room where clients can't relax. Have the room dimmed and possibly a lamp

Endermologie®

with essential oils burning, as often your clinic will have a smell you can't smell and spa music playing. I have lots of plants in my room to also oxygenate. Your treatment table must be comfortable, get on it and try it out for an hour. You don't need to spend heaps of money on a table. Just set up at a height to suit you but at a higher level to save your back. This is also why you need to go to the gym daily to have great core muscles. The room must always be warm. The client is taking off their clothes to start with but also doing endermologie® on a cold client can hurt them or pinch them while breaking down blockages and fat.

These few tips are so important to a successful business and will have your client coming back time and time again. Yes, the treatment and results are important but if the client does not feel at home and can't relax enough to be able to fall asleep during their treatment, then they won't get the best benefits.

Remember, clean! clean! clean! I start work one hour earlier in the morning to sterilise everything and I have a break between each client to sterilise again. Keep your room with no clutter, keep it simple so it doesn't confuse your client; they already have enough going on in their head. Always clean your skirting boards daily and wash floors as your client is constantly face down in their treatment looking at those areas. I have wooden floors so I get the client to leave their shoes on, due to the same hygiene reasons we have for washing our hands with COVID as we sweat from our feet as well.

Payment

I use the Square terminal to take all my payments. It is simple and easy to use and you can pop it in your handbag and take it anywhere. They also have a free booking system included, but I like to use the Acquity booking system as it has a lot of fancier features for your clients. With Acquity, you can do gift vouchers and packages with different treatments using other machines to incorporate a complete ultimate experience.

Pricing treatments is important; the machines are at the top scale in the world to purchase. Don't be afraid of money or asking for it. You have trained years at University and probably still paying off HEC's fees and will be paying high payments in leasing your machine. Be proud of your service to treat clients and charge them accordingly as they are getting the best treatment in the world.

The last tip, don't treat family and friends, it will frustrate you as they won't follow through with their home protocol and don't trade your treatments! You have spent thousands of dollars on your machine, it can end up getting messy on value issues of the treatments.

> 'Success is not final; failure is not fatal: it is the courage to continue that counts.'
> **-Winston Churchill**

CHAPTER 10

New Face Detox

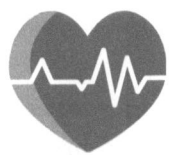

'If you want to succeed you should strike out on new paths, rather than travel the world paths of accepted success.'

-John D. Rockefeller

I just love detoxing! It's a solution for any health issues you have, men and women. Many years ago, I designed up a male stomach protocol at my first clinic in Sanctuary Cove and the distributors were able to pass it onto France LPG to include in their protocols and then onto everyone throughout the world using endermologie®. Now I want to do it again but with the face.

If your clients have chronic fatigue, insomnia, menopause, weight issues causing high blood pressure, auto-immune disease or any health issues, detoxing and learning to swap foods, helps their body to change immediately. Learn how to heal the body, because in reality the client has done this to their body and now it is time to help support them to make changes. Even if it is genes, they have still 'turned their genes on' to give the health issues. These are the words I often say to my clients when they arrive.

I have worked many years on the body detoxing but found I had a missing link, detoxing the face. For this reason, I created a Detox Face protocol to be used in conjunction with the endermolift® treatment. I found being in a coal mine town, everyone is breathing coal dust particles in causing these particles to get embedded in the nasal passages and even cause breathing issues and not being able to get fresh oxygen into our body or worse affect the lungs.

Ask your client, do you have sinus issues? Have you ever checked your nose by blocking one nostril and breathing deep short breaths? Are you blocked? Let your client know this means they are not getting enough oxygen into their body. A lot of us don't breathe properly. Ask, are your ears blocked? Do you feel pressure in your head? Or do your glands get swollen? These are all areas that are giving you warning signs that your client's lymphatic drainage channels in their face are blocking. These are all questions I ask my clients before I start. The endermologie® machine has a whole other side to it that can treat scars, burns, post and pre-operative procedures and most important a new Face Detox protocol by using smaller heads. The treatment is called the endermolift® that is able to go deep within the dermis and increase the hyaluronic acid by 80% to smooth lines, plump and reduce dark circles leaving a glowing complexion. I just love this treatment and have been using it for many years on my face to achieve my high cheekbones and especially for anti-ageing. Also, my clients always talk about their fleshy lips they get from Charlie without even having to use any filler but plumped and natural looking lips!

Blockages

The nasal passages are like another filter system for our body. Funky stuff can get stuck up there such as polyps, parasites, environmental particles and coal dust. I often get clients to do a three day fast on a special tea, with other fluids included. This tea I use has a mixture to help detox parasites, bacteria and mold out of the body. One client blew her nose the third day of her fast and there was a worm that came out of her nose. These little blighters can cause itching in the throat, cough, headaches, sneezing and nasal discharge.

Another way your nose can be clogged is, inflamed blood vessels up inside your nasal passages. This is very common in my clients. The vessels are important as they can help with the flow of the mucus. Living in a mine town, we have huge amounts of dust and are constantly breathing in the particles from coal mining. Air pollution is common everywhere with cars, farming, factories, mining, where particles and gases are suspended in the air and are called aerosols. Then there is the air pollution within the house of mold, lead, asbestos, nitrogen dioxide, radon and carbon monoxide, these can cause symptoms of asthma and allergies.

Allergies are another area that is a huge issue I treat successfully and can be related to air pollution and high histamine. Once we treat the cause of their DNA issues associated with the high histamine, incorporate heaps of plants inside the house to filter the air, flush the channels in the face with endermolift®, the inflamed blood vessels in the nasal passage can repair.

Nasal polyps are also another way of getting nasal blockages. I use a nasal tonic of one drop up each nasal passage with the endermolift® Face Detox protocol to help to clear these away. These polyps are like fleshy tear shaped growths but very important to get out as they cause breathing issues and lack of oxygen to the body. I had a client that was continuously breathing through her mouth. After our session, I got her to sit up and blow her nose and with the tonic and endermolift® protocol, a polyp came out. These polyps can grow back but usually it's to do with health issues going on with the client that need to be addressed.

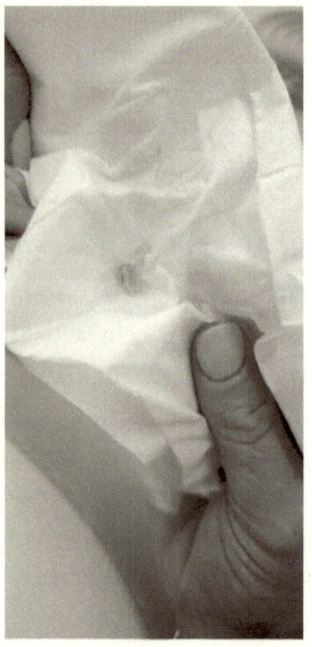

Polyp come out of nasal passage

TMJ or temporomandibular joint is like a hinge connecting your jawbone to your skull and is associated with muscles that can tense up alongside the cheeks that radiate to the sides and top of the head. When you clench or grind your teeth, this can lead to extreme pain and even headaches. A lot of the time you have no idea you are doing this in your sleep. It can be brought on by stress and extreme heavy metal toxicity. The Face Detox protocol includes releasing of the tension and toxins surrounding this area. I was so fortunate to have a client visit me and ask about how I can include this issue in her treatment. With her help we were able to release toxins from this area. The next morning a slight rash came out from the area of the heavy metals and the instant relief was amazing. Being able to finally relieve TMJ also meant it improved joint pain and hip pain that was associated with it. But even more exciting, I was able to include this in my Face Detox protocol.

Step One

First use a good torch to check up the nose for blockages. Also, I like to start with a clean canvas and stop skin particles exfoliating off up into the machine so I do organic scrubs or masks. Try not to use scrubs with large grain particles in them as they will get in the face machine. While applying the scrub, I start a procedure with my fingers to feel where the blockages are in the channels on the face. I focus on the channel from the eye duct to the top of the ear. Then the eye duct to below the ear, using deep circular motions. I also do it below the ear, to release the lymph system for drainage down into the throat and to check the nodes aren't blocked. Then the final two channels are from the side of the nose to the middle of the ear and the side of the nose to below the ear. The movements are small, circular and deep, to promote blood flow but always checking to see where the areas are blocked and where I need to focus on with the endermolift® Face Detox treatment.

I finish with a hot towel cleanse and most importantly, I also go over with a tissue to cleanse of any particles of the scrub or mask. I apply a nourishing cream, not an oil as it makes the skin too slippery and we need to get deep into the tissue. This also allows you to double check with your fingers to see if there are any grains of the scrub left on the face. I use a towel to whisk these away. If you find you are no good at getting all the particles of the skin use a mask instead of a scrub but remember it needs to be two of them.

I then use my nasal tonic of ½-1 drop up each nasal passage while holding the other nasal closed. I get the client to take short deep breaths in as it gently melts the blockages and pushes the tonic and blockages through the passages and eventually down to the throat. Make sure when it hits the throat that you get the client to do a couple more short breaths, just to move it through. I highly recommend this nasal tonic as it is an important part of the treatment and you need all components to make the treatment work. Please see the back of the book for more information on the specialised tonic used to purchase.

Step Two

Next, I use the firming setting on the Face Detox protocol. I use the ergolift® treatment head to drain the neck upwards and across as exactly on the endermolift® machine protocol, giving a neck lift at the same time. I make sure I tuck in under the jawline, as nearly everyone has blockages here. You can see most clients have a puffy area here. It's important to move it, so their face is more chiselled in a man and more defined in a woman.

While doing this release, I focus on the nodes under the ears with small circular moves and then from the ears down the side of the neck into the middle of the bottom of the neck. This allows the client to have a clearway for them to swallow the gunk that flows down. It's really neat! The next morning, the clients often find their stools are shiny and have excess mucus in them from this procedure. You can see when you are clearing this passage as your client will start to swallow and you can see and feel lumps of mucus being dislodged and swallowed down the throat. Depending on the client, if there are thyroid issues, I will also include flushing very gently over the thyroid with butterfly like movements.

Step three

The next method we achieve is to move backwards in our procedure so that there are no blockages and all the channels are unblocked by the time we get to the nasal passages. Therefore, the next procedure we follow is using the same protocol as in the endermolift® machine doing the jawline. The moves are upward and then across.

Then I add my release technique again for the nodes under the ear doing small slow circular moves. You will be able to feel lumps that are the blockages here. It is important to drain not too hard, as it can be painful if you press hard down. Often you can feel clients that have had a virus in the past, the nodes can feel congested as the body has tried to fight it but still storing the virus in the tissue. I move up to the middle of the ear again with small circular moves. I then link both these moves up and follow through again with the original endermolift® protocol.

Step Four

The next step is the nasal and cheek bone lift. Using the same protocol again as the endermolift® face machine, I warm the cheek up to give a nice face-lift with cheekbone definition. By this time if the tonic did not move down the throat at the beginning it sure will be now, breaking up the blockages. The client is often swallowing huge chunks of gunk coming down from the nasal, eyes, ear and lymph channels.

This next step starts on the first side of the nostril and drains to the middle of the ear. You can feel the blockages start to drain. Then the next channel to clear is from the nostril to below the ear lobe. It is important to do both directions as sometimes the blockages won't dislodge and this movement helps to flush them through. Continue to drain from ear to throat.

Step Five

This next step is the forehead and is again following the similar protocol as the endermolift® face treatment on the machine, but also includes circular motions on the side of the temples. This move helps to release tension and help with headaches associated with it. Include a drain from the bottom of the eyes back up to the side of the temple helping to drain the sinus again but also giving an eye lift. Under the eyes are delicate tissues and the forehead move is the only time you can use it as you will notice the change in the movement of the flaps. Often under the eyes it darkens due to the blockages. The forehead is drained in all two directions, upwards to the hairline and across to the temples.

Step Six

Now we change to the butterfly smaller head on the ergolift® treatment head and using the same endermolift® protocol on the machine, but this time including the eye ducts. A lot of clients are blocked around this area and often you can see their eyelids are darkened, puffy and swollen. Start with the eyelids to drain towards the top of the ear, making sure you get in close to the eye duct. Then the next move is amazing, it's going up on the inside of the eye over the eye duct with gentle butterfly moves to help drain the eye and promote healthy blood flow. Include again under the eye to tighten and drain the tissue that causes those awful bags and darkening with blockages.

Step Seven

Changing to TR30 head I use this next step to help release locked jaw, grinding and clenching of teeth. This area is your temporomandibular TMJ that can cause headaches, dizziness, nausea and even muscle soreness. We can store a lot of emotion in this area due to stress and anxiety. The move needs to be light pressure starting on 1 to 2 level. Some of the releases I've had from clients in this final move have been outstanding. I work gently behind the lower ear lobe releasing in circular motions and finish off with sliding up the base of the neck to behind the ear and from the base of the neck to in front of the ear.

These steps are easy to follow and the results are huge. I do not use this treatment on children. My results and experiences with my clients and their changes in using this Face protocol have been amazing.

Please don't worry if you are a visual learner as I have a link in the back of the book to learn this protocol online.

'Never be afraid to try something new because life gets boring when you stay within the limits of what you already know'

-Anonymous

CHAPTER 11

Machine Combinations

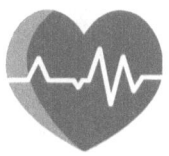

'Machines take me by surprise with great frequency'
-Alan Turing

I spoke about machine combinations throughout the book so I thought it would be important to devote a chapter to other machines you can bring in and combine to make your treatments the 'Ultimate Worx' experience. It's all about getting the best result for your client to improve their health, so they get that wow factor experience. Endermologie® and endermolift® is that wow factor but now we just want to push it to the next level.

My Ultimate Worx experience includes a Foot Detox, One Hour endermologie®, Infra-Red Wrap and endermolift® face-detox. Also, if you do the five-day detox programme it can take you to the next holistic level as it also includes the sound therapy.

Endermologie®

As a therapist if you are new to endermologie® you will need to slowly build up to do one-hour treatment, as it can be very tiring on the body. It took me a good 6-8 months before I had the physical strength to do the hour treatments as each treatment can be a work-out on your body. Start out with 30 minutes and slowly build up to the hour. The hour endermologie® is amazing. The client instantly relaxes and often falls asleep on the second round up their spine to release the toxins and spinal fluid into the brain. It is the ultimate experience, the secret to your client that will keep them coming back again and again to improve their health. Clients not only need a change in their health but they are always looking for a way to relax and reduce stress.

Foot Detox

The first machine I want to discuss and is very popular out here in the mines is the foot detox. I love this machine. It's so fascinating to watch all the heavy metals come out of the feet. This little beauty purges heavy metals, yeast, parasites, reduces inflammation, enhances the immune system and reduces your acid in your body. I love it when the parasites come out, especially when you get the long tapeworms. There are a variety of foot detox machines, some work on different levels to give you stronger or less detox from the feet. There are some from overseas that I wouldn't use due to the safety issues. I have designed my machines up from a Doctor in the USA in 1999 and over the years have tweaked my machines internally to achieve my desired outcomes, foremost of eliminating parasites and heavy metals, as coal dust. The technology has changed so much with the foot detox over the years. The old versions or some of the current overseas versions do not use the positive and negative ionization.

The quality of the arrays are important as like any machine using good quality parts is important. I have designed a machine up from using the shell off other machines and then changing the insides to accommodate what I need to pull out, such as coal dust, parasites, yeast and candida. It has taken me years to get to this stage as none of the machines online were able to do this. I hope to be able to sell these machines to therapists very soon as they are strong to use and very beneficial in your clients results for detoxing.

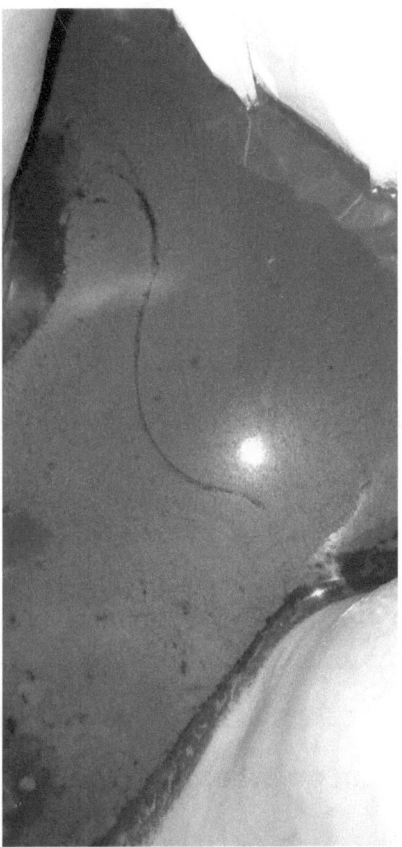

Massive tapeworm

I have included a picture of a client that had a massive tapeworm come out, that is common. Her whole health changed after we completed the foot detox. The die-off effect or the parasite poo, from pulling one of these tapeworms out; can make the client feel very sick but with the following combination of the other machines, the die-off effect was minimal and that's one of the reasons I love to combine machines.

Endermologie®

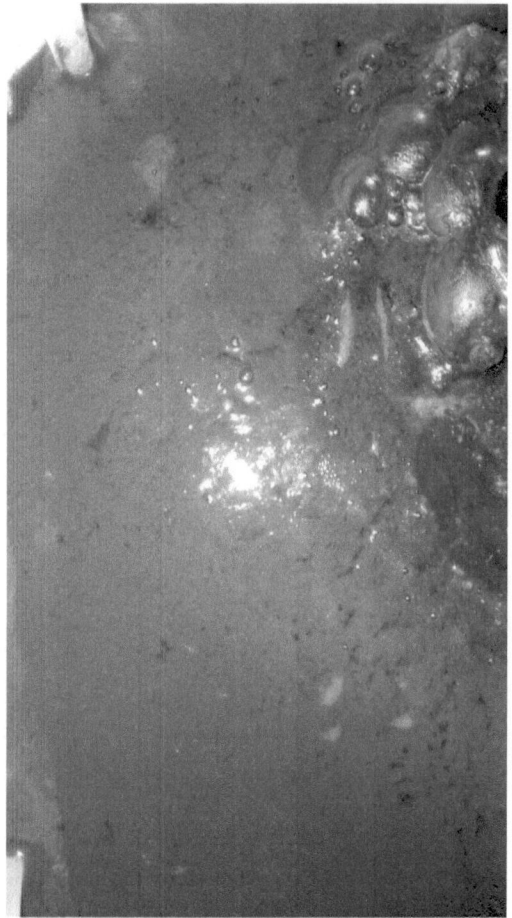

Cream parasites from Foot Detox

I also use a 'pulling technique' in the foot detox, I was privileged to learn from being on a Vision Quest with a Cherokee Indian lady many years ago in the USA. I learnt how to draw or pull-on clients detoxing to enhance it, to move more toxins through. The secret to a successful clinical foot detox is learning this process of drawing on the client and using a specialised machine. I have many clients travel for miles to see me, as one treatment of this machine can change their health immediately. However, I always combine it with another due to the die-off effect.

Machine Combinations

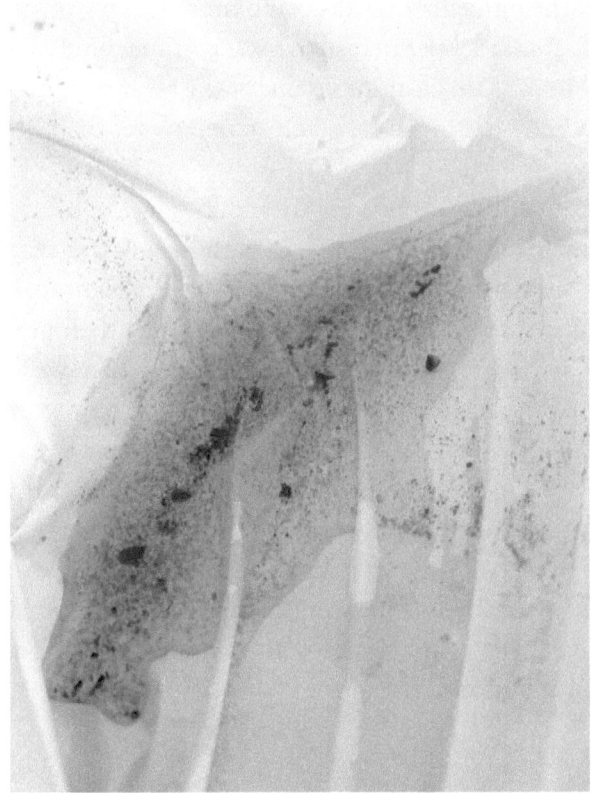

Coal dust particles removed

It is amazing to see when I tip out the bucket all the coal dust left in the bottom as per picture provided. Sometimes especially underground miners, their feet and legs get a dull ache as the coal dust particles are large and drain out through the feet and can be quite sharp.

Practically all my clients out here in Moranbah get the Moranbah blue in their foot detox. It is this fluorescent blue that floats on top of the foot detox. It is a side effect of living in a mine town, but the great thing is we can live here in a healthy state as long as we detox. I find clients can get very confused with brain fog, memory loss, lack of concentration, when they have heavy metal toxicity in their body. I like to use this machine if the client is feeling down, fatigued or just not happy. The immediate results combining with the other machines is amazing. As stated before, I don't use this machine on its own as much now because to clear toxins out of the head to improve mental health, the body has to have a detox as well to get the full benefit.

Detoxing the children out here in Moranbah I absolutely love it! They line up for their foot detox from early ages as 3-4 years old. The changes in their behaviour later on is incredible. They are happy, less angry and a lot calmer. The wee little ones also let their parents know when they are ready for another one. They say, "Can we see Ms Fee again!" I love to teach them how to feel good and know when it is time for their next one. A lot of parents are putting so many supplements into their children these days. It's not good for their body as it can store in their tissue and you really don't know if you're overdosing and that is so dangerous. Instead, the most important part for a child out here in Moranbah, is to detox the toxins out, so when they eat a healthy meal their body absorbs all the nutrients naturally rather than constantly supplementing.

Infra-Red Wrap/Straps

My next favourite combination machine that is always followed after the endermologie® treatment is the infra-red wrap or straps as the men call it. I use this machine to compliment the endermologie® or foot detox to double flush out everything I have broken up within the treatment. After the endermologie®, clients need to exercise but they are so relaxed they don't feel like doing any. We need to push the toxins out of the body. This machine is from Germany. It promotes the client to have a good sweat internally. It's not the normal everyday sweat from the outside of the skin that tries to cool the body down. The infra-red rays penetrate the skin 1-2 inches and promote excess blood circulation that then promotes the lymph system to kick into gear. It is similar to a 10km run, while you are lying down.

Machine Combinations

I am sorry to say, it's not available anymore. I used to use an infra-red ray sauna but couldn't get the rays into the tissue to repair but I love them for a great healthy sweat. Great news though! I have sourced a similar machine in the USA and is available if you would like to invest in one with similar results but they are very costly. The important issue with infra-red rays is to get one that you can wrap with silicone bandages onto the tissue as infra-red rays need to penetrate the tissue to benefit. Beware of the ones from overseas that the rays are not the correct temperature and actually are not an infra-red ray.

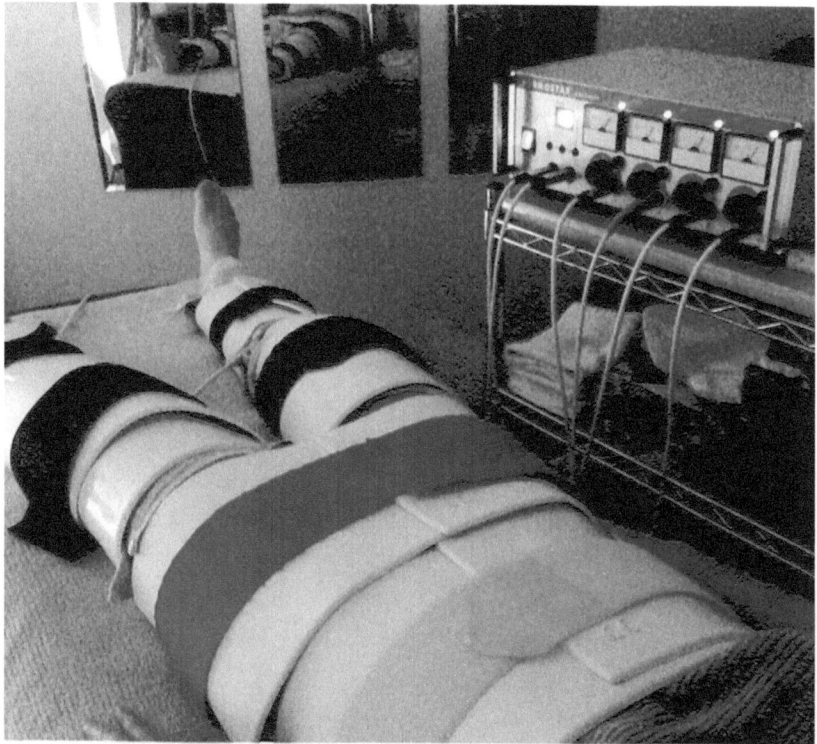

Chilling in the straps wrap

This wrap uses infra-red rays to penetrate the inner layers of the skin and helps to heal degenerative tissues, muscles and bone but most importantly flush toxic inflammatory conditions. It also promotes a flushing in the skin that is great for viral, bacterial and fungi toxins in the body or issues with rashes. This is done through the balance in the temperature of the infra-red rays.

I have used this machine for clients returning from overseas with health infections on their skin and had amazing results. Within 1-2 sessions, the infection is gone. Or one of my favourite ailments to treat is an inflammatory sore back included with the Ultimate Worx treatments. A lot of lower back issues can be the kidneys with kidney stones. I often have clients' backs heal completely after we reduce the stones and move through with changed lifestyle habits. I also use it for colds, the flu, pleurisy, bronchitis and pneumonia infusing the rays directly into the lungs. The healing process is three times quicker as it flushes out the inflammation and promotes blood flow to the organ to help heal quickly. Your body needs to be flushed as we can become stagnant with toxins in our body and inflamed areas won't heal. I often call this wrap, the happy wrap as after it you feel as if a load has come off your back. You actually feel lighter.

Face-Detox

The following treatment while the client is in the wrap is the Face Detox. As stated earlier, I use a herbal remedy I have designed this herbal tonic mix to snort up the nostrils to remove blockages such as; coal dust, parasites, polyps and all sorts of blockages. I have a link to order this tonic at the end of the book. The most important process is the drainage technique I have designed up. This I have released to you in chapter 10. The results are amazing. Our environment these days is not only causing our body to accumulate toxins but also our eyes, ears and nasal passages to block.

Sound Therapy

This section I have left till last. It is my area I have just fallen in love with without even searching for it. I was invited to a taste of Sound Therapy at a two-day workshop and was so fascinated that I went on a journey of more intense training with some amazing sound masters and took from each one of them and designed my own techniques. I would love to take you on this journey of healing, transformation, and calming with Tibetan Sound Therapy course. To teach you how to heal your clients of all their emotional and mental blockages.

Our spiritual aspect of ourselves can get blocked. You can physically remove blockages in the body of lumps and bumps but if there are mental and emotional issues blocking your client, the conditions will keep coming back. Your cells are affected with how we think and react to everyday life and situations through our memories. It is about letting go of these stuck, stagnant memories that we can push down inside us to cause our blockages.

Sometimes we are not even aware we have them, until a disease starts within our body and it's related to stress. Stress can destroy the body; adrenal fatigue can destroy the body. If you can't stop and truly relax and go into a meditative state, something is going on inside you to cause this. Sound Therapy finds your blockages and releases them, it is so soothing that often my client's go under into a deep meditative state.

There are two types of bowls available; the Tibetan bowls and the crystal bowls. The true Tibetan bowls are made in Nepal with seven metals hammered into one alloy while the modern ones are made by a machine from tin and copper and sound beautiful but the true bowls are a majestic sound. I love the Tibetan bowls as they are very grounding and earthy, bringing us back to our roots. The second type of bowels are the crystal bowls that are made of a quartz crystal but some are also made from different crystals such as amethyst and rose. They are new and have been approximately around since 1990 and are great for balancing your chakras or energy in your body. It is a personal preference as to which ones you use or even both.

I am so excited to now have a course for you to learn the bowls as a therapist or even as a client. It is important to be trained in these bowls as the vibration on an organ or body can be very strong.

There are many more machines out there that will be ideal for you to include in your business. The most important part of owning a machine is the research, not from just the manufacturer but from outside interests to check the machine is true to what it can do and most importantly, you have a passion for it. Your passion is what makes a successful business. My happy smile and my genuine passion to help heal my clients to become healthier and happier is what I live for!!!

Machine Combinations

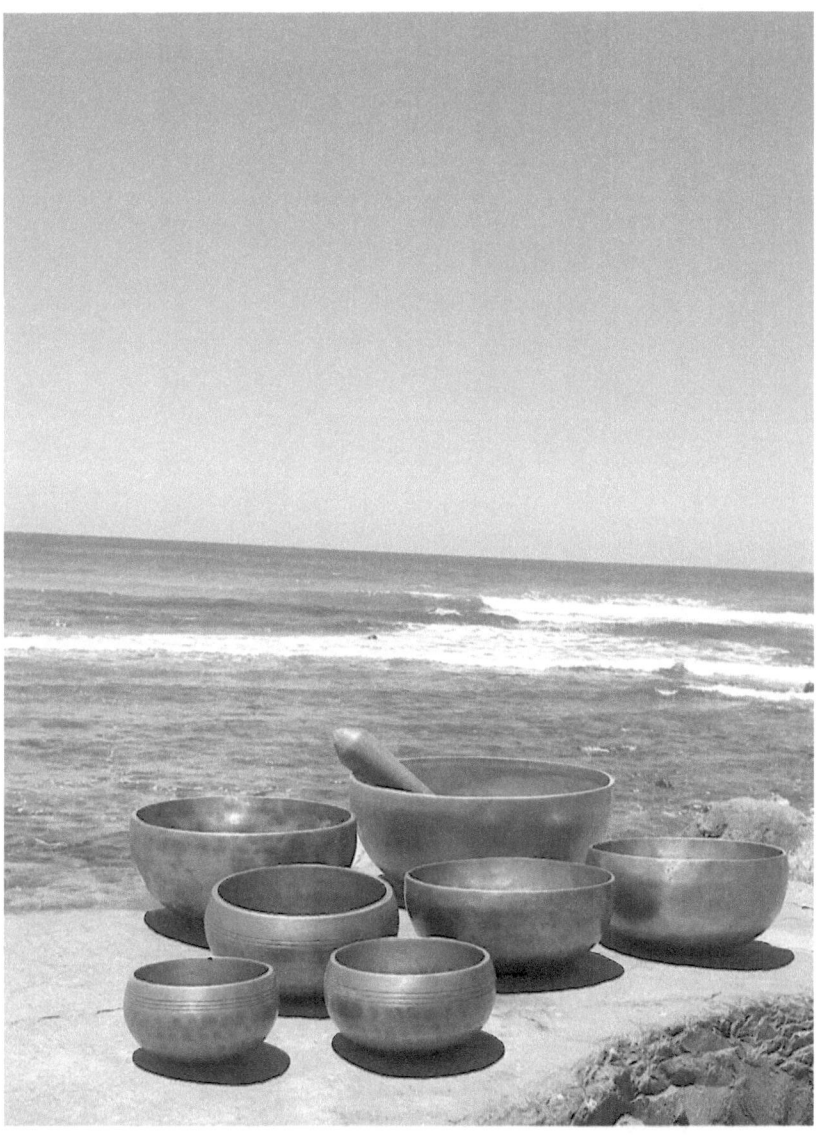

'My clients are more than my clients, they are my friends and family'

Fee Selby

SUMMARY

Part Two

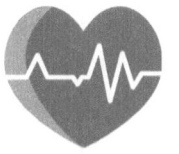

'Opportunities don't happen. You create them'
-Chris Grosser

Endermologie® is a passion, a dream I have been doing to help as many clients as possible achieve their dreams of the ultimate healthy mind and healthy body. From the time the client comes in to see me for their first treatment when they are tired, fatigued and fed up with their job and home life, till after one to four treatments when their health, state of mind has improved and they are coping at work and connecting with their family again. The inches melt off their body, in areas they have never been able to lose, helping their health issues improve.

Endermologie® can sculpt the body into a fit, lean, flexible body, removing visceral fat surrounding the muscle and organs. Don't let your clients be a statistic of excess subcutaneous fat stored under

Endermologie®

their skin all over their body causing excess body fluid, resulting in blockages and causing them fatigue. The visceral fat that is collecting around the liver, pancreas, intestines is affecting how the hormones in their body function and is dangerous. Or even worse, leaving this fat too long increases the risk of heart problems and many health issues such as diabetes.

Don't let your client become a statistic of ill health needing constant medication, or operations to cut their body open. Learn to pivot their health into 2021 and beat all the odds. Have a healthy lifestyle and mindset so that anything is possible for your client to achieve their goals. These are the words I feed to my clients. These are the words you will pass onto your clients to project into a successful, healthy business of healing so many people that are going to follow you, no matter where you move to. I have clients that still travel hundreds of miles out west to see me for my five-day packages, to reboot their systems, to reboot their health. Find your passion in endermologie® to pivot forward into 2021.

Leave the year of the pandemic behind with a big kick up the arse! Take from it the importance of your own and clients health and how quickly it can change everyone's life, if you don't look after your body. Remember you can always be busy earning an income but if your body gets sick, no amount of money can cure it…

> 'To ensure good health: eat lightly, breathe deeply, live moderately, cultivate cheerfulness and maintain an interest in life'
>
> **-William Londen**

Part Two

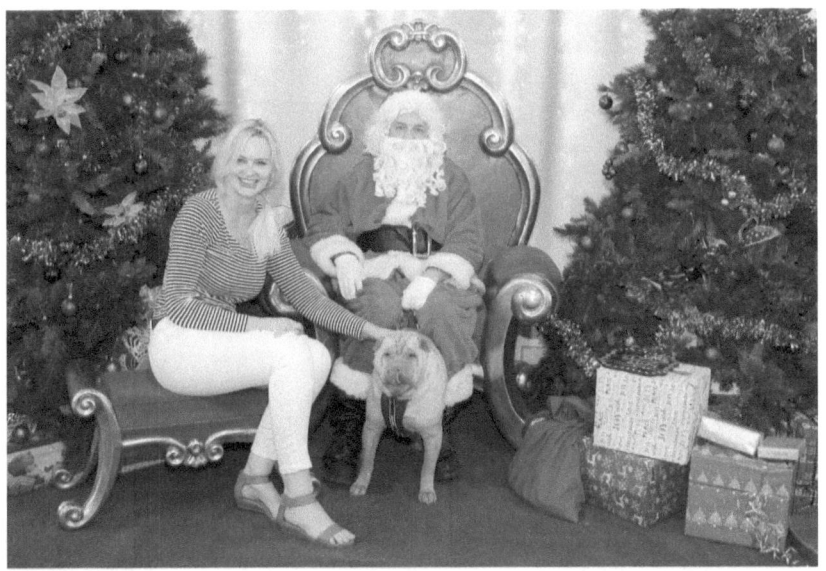

Fee and her receptionist Brandy

About the Author

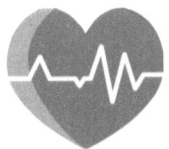

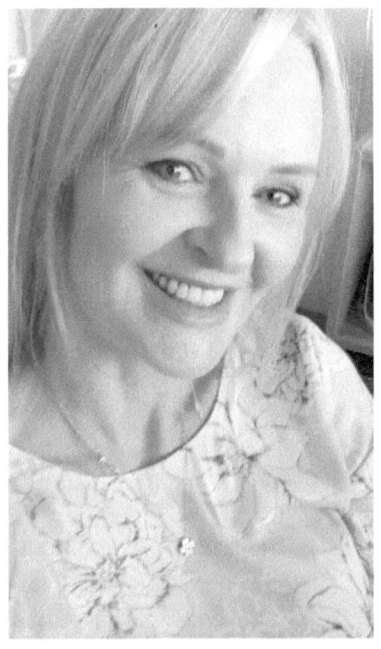

As everyone calls her, Fee grew up in New Zealand, always remembering her mother and sister having weight issues and seeing the pain they went through to try to combat it. As a child, she kept to herself a lot as she could know what people were thinking and feeling. It was such a challenge to try to block it out as a child. Often, she would have spirit come and visit her when she was so young and hated it as it made her sensitive to the people around her. As she got older, she tried to block it until she had a terrible car accident she went through to the light. It was the most incredible experience with God she has ever had, and there are no words for it. Fee remembers being told to go back, you need to heal others and to remember we are all the same but in different bodies and our experiences have shaped who we are, but in the end, we are all the same. The next minute she was being dragged out of the car by a doctor on the way to the hospital. This was such a coincidental occurrence as it was a remote country road. This was why Fee started on her journey over 30 years ago to heal as many people as possible. God had another plan for Fee.

Fee was drawn to Australia for the warmth and beautiful beaches and moved over to the Gold Coast when she was 18 years old. She started as a beauty therapist and quickly expanded into owning the top prestige clinic at Sanctuary Cove that won Day Spa/Clinic of the Year, Customer Excellence of the Year and introduced the journey of endermologie®. Fee has two very successful children Manuel and Anastasia with three grandchildren Sid, London and Georgie.

Sadly, Fee got melanoma twice and later divorced after going through a marriage with alcoholism and DV. It was a low time in her life, but this helped her to project more in-depth into the health industry and find answers to cancer and specialising in mental health issues such as alcoholism, schizophrenia, depression, anxiety and bipolar.

Fee returned back out west to Moranbah, a coal mine town that she was drawn to for her fascination in detoxing coal. Here she learnt every aspect of detoxing coal out of the miners and designed up programmes for clients that travel all over Australia to come and see her for chronic fatigue, autoimmune diseases, cancer, tumours, weight issues to name a few, that experience a 5-day intense programme on her machines, herbal tonics, teas, sound therapy and DNA. The results are excellent, and her lifetime friendships are even more memorable.

Fiona was honoured to receive a scholarship to the Bond University for the Bachelor of Communication majoring in Public Relations and Human Interaction focusing on her Aboriginal studies that lead to the honour of being taught women's issues by two Aboriginal Elders.

About the Author

Fee then went on to further studies to become a Naturopath, Western Herbalist and a Nutritionist.

In her younger years, she studied Psychosynthesis Psychology and a Diploma in Counselling. She has completed the Hoffman Process and walked the Kokoda trail in PNG.

Fee has studied with many great mentors, travelling around the world to many workshops such as such as Tony Robbins and Mathew Hussey.

Fee's passion for science led her to become one of the top DNA analysts, that can test all your genes to find out what potential or current issues you have going on in your brain and body and the most exciting part to be able to correct.

Fee loves yoga, meditation and the gym with her favourite pastime, riding her old Harley Davidson out to the Nebo bush pub for a counter lunch. She loves hiking in the bush and wishes one day to get a houseboat and cruise the waterways or an RV van to visit all parts of Australia.

Fee's passion for the future is to renovate her miner's cottage she currently brought for her clinic, and continue to treat as many clients as possible to free them of disease in their bodies and teach them how to use her programmes to keep healthy. Fee believes we don't need to go on crazy diets, have dangerous surgeries or over supplementing, just eat normally by swapping foods and teach our body to get rid of the waste, so we don't block up. Also, to bring up healthy children that won't carry on the generations of diseases passed through our DNA.

Fee's other passion is to teach practitioners in endermologie® the benefits and knowledge that she has received over the many years practising, so endermologie® will be treated on as many clients as possible.

References

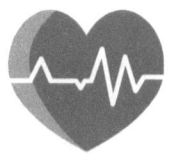

2020 Australian Institute of Health and Welfare. *Children with mental illness.* www.aihw.gov.au. Australian Government.

2014 Barcley, Rachel *Not just the ovaries: your brain makes estrogen too.* Healthline. www.healthline.com

2020 Davis, Tchiki Ph.D *What is the COMT gene and how does it affect your health?* Psychology Today. www.psychologytoday.com

2010 Dr David L Watts *Trace Elements and other essential Nutrients*, writer's B-L-O-C-K

2011 Galvin, K. Bishop M. *Case Studies for Complementary therapists a collaborate approach.* Elsevier Australia.

2020 Kuester Dr Victoria. *Growing bones, growing concerns: A guide to growth plates.* Children's Hospital of Richmond at VCU. www.chrichmond.org

2019 Mercola, Joseph. *The damaging effects of Oxalates on the body.* Mercola take control of your health newsletter. www.articles.mercola.com

2020 Murrell, Daniel. *Low and normal blood oxygen levels: what to know.* Medical news today. www.medicalnewstoday.com

2020 Patricia, Cohen. *Judge Puts Cloud Over Settlement. Of Roundup Cancer Claims.* The New York Times. Wwwnytimes.com

2020 Preston ND, Cynthia. *When estrogen becomes a problem.* www.drprestonnd.com

2018 Pizzorno, Dr J, Toxins – *Primary Drivers of Chronic Disease with Dr Joseph Pizzorno.* Integria Symposium Healthcare)

2016 Schwartz, Larry. *7 Types of Plastic Wreaking on Our Health.*www.ecowatch.com

2003 Tomporowski, Phillip. *Effects of acute bouts of exercise on cognition.* www.pubmed.gov.

2008 University of Cincinnati. *Plastic bottles release potentially harmful chemicals (Bisphenol A) after contact with hot liquids.* www.sciencedaily.com

2018 Whelan, Corey. *Lactic Acidosis: What you need to know.* Healthline. www.healthline.com

Offers

Free Sound Therapy

A free Sound Therapy recorded session for you to listen to just before bed or when you are feeling stressed, to help relax and rejuvenate the mind. These bowls are also excellent for your child in helping them relax and sleep soundly.

This free Sound Therapy recording is setting up the foundational groundwork to relax, rejuvenate and release stuck emotional junk in your nervous system and your cells.

If you find them as healing as much as I do-follow the link to take it to the next level to become a certified Sound Therapist and start your own business.
fionaselby.net

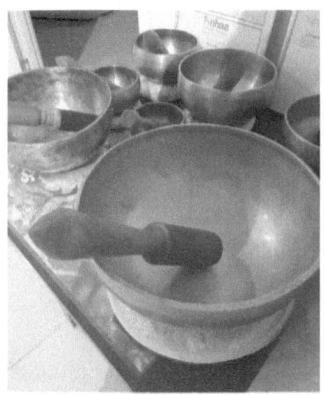

Face Detox Protocol for Therapists

If you are confident with the Face Detox protocol in chapter 10 below is the link to purchase the herbal remedy. I have designed to snort up the nostrils to remove blockages such as; coal dust, parasites, polyps and all sorts of blockages only to use in conjunction with the Face Detox protocol. This is for therapists only.
fionaselby.net

Or learn easily the new protocol for the Face Detox, recorded for your convenience.

I will take you through step by step the protocol you need to include in your business for detoxing the face.

The most important process is the drainage technique I have designed up. The results are amazing. Our environment these days is not only causing our body to accumulate toxins but also our eyes, ears and nasal passages to block.
http://fionaselby.net

The Ultimate 5-day Retreat

Book a 5-day personalised one on one Ultimate package retreat to change your life.

This is for clients that need to seriously change their health or need a huge push into getting a healthy mind and healthy body back to optimal health. I will personally take you through your five days and transform your health. This is not a group package but a individualised programme for each client.

Living remotely is a huge part of the success in this package as there are no distractions while you are here, you are totally focused.

Offers

You are required to complete the four-hour treatments daily involving four machines; the endermologie® foot detox, infra-ray wrap, face detox and the sound bowls. Then your package also includes healthy food meals, herbal tonics, herbal teas, meditation, yoga, swimming and PT sessions.

My Ultimate Experience Retreat is your path to your freedom to a healthy body and a healthy mind. Whether it's chronic fatigue, thyroid issues, infertility, anxiety, depression or gaining control of your weight, it's your next step to freedom to a healthy body at last. I will walk you through step-by-step in making those changes that are baby steps and so easy to achieve. This package involves you stepping up each day to make changes in your health. Never have to diet again. Let me take you on your endermologie® path to the secret, to look good, feel good and achieve the 'Wow' factor.

http://fionaselby.net

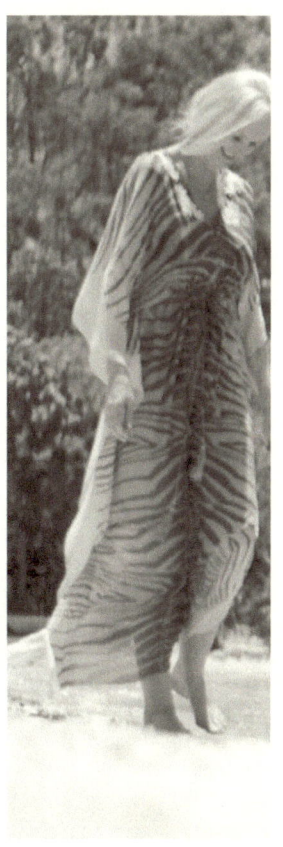

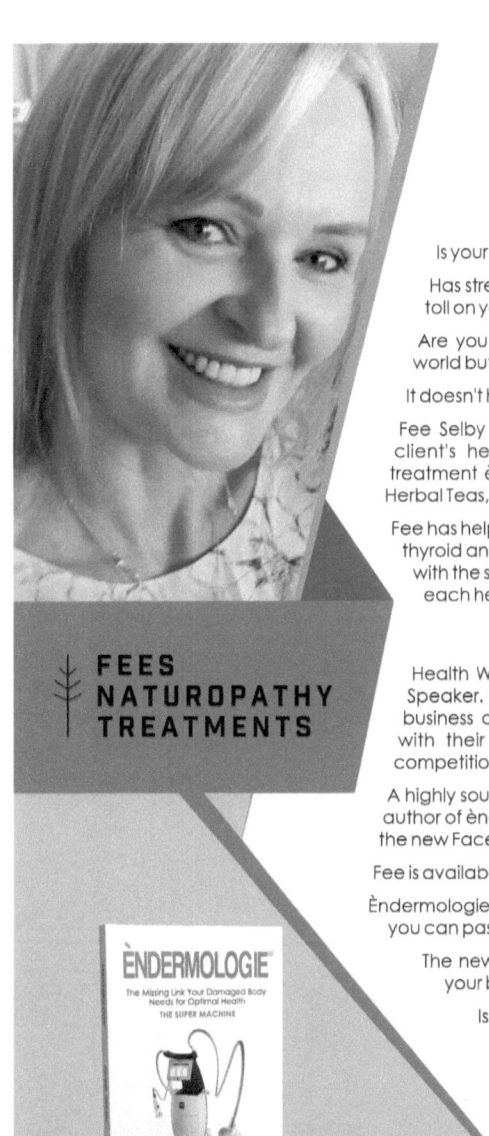

FEE SELBY

THE CHALLENGE TODAY:

Is your body tired, run down and diseased?

Has stress, anxiety, weight gain and depression taken its toll on your life?

Are you fed up with pills and potions that promise the world but leave you frustrated and with no results?

It doesn't have to be that way.

Fee Selby reveals her successful 30 years of treating her client's health issues with a super machine using the treatment èndermologie® DNA, Herbal Tonics, specialised Herbal Teas, Swap Food Protocol and Sound Therapy!

Fee has helped clients with anxiety, depression, menopause, thyroid and weight issues, completely heal their bodies and with the successful èndermologie® protocols used to treat each health issue.

WHAT PEOPLE ARE SAYING...

Health Wealth Strategist, Mental Health and Weight-loss Speaker. Fee Selby helps organizations, professionals and business owners create and achieve outstanding results with their clientele that differentiates them from their competition and increases their bottom line.

A highly sought after professional speaker, Fee is a published author of èndermologie® the super machine and designer of the new Face Detox protocol.

Fee is available for speaking/training on the following topics...

Èndermologie® and all its aspects in health and achievements you can pass onto your clientele.

The new Face Protocol and the benefits it can bring to your business.

Issues on real life struggles of weight issues, thyroid, anxiety, depression, menopause, children's health and men's health in our toxic environments with all her valuable knowledge of treating in a coal mine town and the tools available to give you the advantage in changing your health to an optimal healthy lifestyle.

If you want to invite Fee Selby as a Guest Speaker at your event email us at feeselby@yahoo.com
BOOK FEE TODAY!

FEES NATUROPATHY TREATMENTS

As seen on: Professional Beauty Magazine, The Gold Coast Bulletin

Notes

Endermologie®

Notes

Endermologie®

Notes

www.ingramcontent.com/pod-product-compliance
Lightning Source LLC
Chambersburg PA
CBHW021440080526
44588CB00009B/610